NEW DEVELOPMENTS IN MEDICAL RESEARCH

VITAL SIGNS

AN OVERVIEW

NEW DEVELOPMENTS IN MEDICAL RESEARCH

Additional books and e-books in this series can be found on Nova's website under the Series tab.

NEW DEVELOPMENTS IN MEDICAL RESEARCH

VITAL SIGNS

AN OVERVIEW

ROY ABI ZEID DAOU
AND
JOSEF BÖRCSÖK
EDITORS

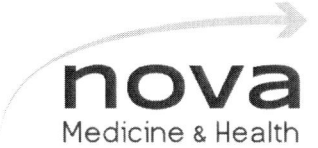

Copyright © 2020 by Nova Science Publishers, Inc.

All rights reserved. No part of this book may be reproduced, stored in a retrieval system or transmitted in any form or by any means: electronic, electrostatic, magnetic, tape, mechanical photocopying, recording or otherwise without the written permission of the Publisher.

We have partnered with Copyright Clearance Center to make it easy for you to obtain permissions to reuse content from this publication. Simply navigate to this publication's page on Nova's website and locate the "Get Permission" button below the title description. This button is linked directly to the title's permission page on copyright.com. Alternatively, you can visit copyright.com and search by title, ISBN, or ISSN.

For further questions about using the service on copyright.com, please contact:
Copyright Clearance Center
Phone: +1-(978) 750-8400 Fax: +1-(978) 750-4470 E-mail: info@copyright.com.

NOTICE TO THE READER

The Publisher has taken reasonable care in the preparation of this book, but makes no expressed or implied warranty of any kind and assumes no responsibility for any errors or omissions. No liability is assumed for incidental or consequential damages in connection with or arising out of information contained in this book. The Publisher shall not be liable for any special, consequential, or exemplary damages resulting, in whole or in part, from the readers' use of, or reliance upon, this material. Any parts of this book based on government reports are so indicated and copyright is claimed for those parts to the extent applicable to compilations of such works.

Independent verification should be sought for any data, advice or recommendations contained in this book. In addition, no responsibility is assumed by the Publisher for any injury and/or damage to persons or property arising from any methods, products, instructions, ideas or otherwise contained in this publication.

This publication is designed to provide accurate and authoritative information with regard to the subject matter covered herein. It is sold with the clear understanding that the Publisher is not engaged in rendering legal or any other professional services. If legal or any other expert assistance is required, the services of a competent person should be sought. FROM A DECLARATION OF PARTICIPANTS JOINTLY ADOPTED BY A COMMITTEE OF THE AMERICAN BAR ASSOCIATION AND A COMMITTEE OF PUBLISHERS.

Additional color graphics may be available in the e-book version of this book.

Library of Congress Cataloging-in-Publication Data

ISBN: 978-1-53617-765-7

Published by Nova Science Publishers, Inc. † New York

Contents

Preface   vii

Introduction   ix

Chapter 1   The Effects of Exercise Training on Blood Pressure among Adults   1
Mohammed Ali Fakhro, Rim Fayad and Fatima Al Ameen

Chapter 2   The Effect of Surgical Stress on Vital Signs and Nursing Care   15
Selda Mert Boğa and Aylin Aydin Sayilan

Chapter 3   Prediction and Detection of Epilepsy Seizures Using Electrophysiological Measurements   27
Nashaat El Halabi, Roy Abi Zeid Daou, Roger Achkar, Ali Hayek and Josef Boercsoek

Chapter 4   Safer Drug Administration via Smart Syringe Pump Using Patient's Monitor Feedback   81
Hasnaa ElKheshen, Ibrahim Deni, Alaa Baalbaky, Saeed H. Bamashmos, Mohamad Dib, Lara Hamawy, Mohamad Hajj-Hassan, Mohamad Abou Ali and Abdallah Kassem

Chapter 5	Implementation of a Monitoring System that Notifies Healthcare Providers of a Sudden Medical Emergency Occurring to a Driver *Joseph Khattar, Carla Zeine, Roy Abi Zeid Daou, Ali Hayek and Josef Boercsoek*	**107**
Chapter 6	Structural and Functional Abnormalities in Major Depressive Disorder *Lara Hamawy, Ahmed Alnaggar, Khaled Omais, Mohamad Abou Ali, Mohamad Hajj-Hassan and Abdallah Kassem*	**131**
About the Editors		**161**
Index		**163**

PREFACE

As defined by *Medical Plus encyclopedia*, Vital signs reflect essential body functions, including your heartbeat, breathing rate, temperature, and blood pressure. Your health care provider may watch, measure, or monitor your vital signs to check your level of physical functioning.

Another coherent definition was also presented by *Merriam-Webster dictionary* stating that the vital signs are simply defined as being the *signs of life*.

Going back to the main vital signs, they are no common determination for these parameters: some references indicate that they are four, others five or even seven. However, almost all the references mentioned that the *Body Temperature*, the *Pulse Rate*, the *Respiration Rate*, and the *Blood Pressure* are the essential vital signs.

Nevertheless, all previous studies highlight the importance of monitoring the vital signs ratios in order to get a healthier life style. Thus, a good monitoring and control of these parameters will probably reduce the risks of health problems and yield to a better life style.

This book focuses, not only on the novel approaches to measure the vital signs and their effects of the physical activities on these ratios, but proposes some engineering-based applications in order to integrate the measurement of these parameters in innovative systems.

INTRODUCTION

This book is based on six chapters which are mainly related to the vital signs and their integration in several applications and measurements.

The first chapter presents a review over the effects of exercise training on the blood pressure level among adults. Although the link between physical activity and risks of cardiovascular disease and premature mortality is proposed, a particular importance is attributed to the reduction in the frequency of physical inactivity that will be considered as one of the nine global targets to improve the prevention and treatment of non-communicable diseases.

The second chapter shows the effect of surgical stress on vital signs and nursing care. Despite the need of a surgery to save someone's life, neuro-endocrine responses occur while waiting in the preoperative period. This phase can result in physiological changes in vital signs, including elevated heart and respiratory rates and blood pressure, and pain. All these changes will be treated in this chapter.

The third chapter proposes a novel approach for prediction and detection of epilepsy seizures using electrophysiological measurements. The EEG and the ECG systems are used to record and analyze the cardiac and the brain physiological. Based on these recording and while using several artificial intelligence-based algorithms, the system will be able to predict and detect any seizure that will occur/occurs to the epileptic patient.

The fourth chapter presents an integrated system of a smart syringe pump with a patient monitor's readings. The main objective of this system is to limit human errors caused by nurses that must manual decrease the flow-rate of the drug delivered to the patient as for the case of stage two hypertensive patients. The proposed system can be considered as an advance step towards a fully automated treatment and monitoring patients in the intensive care environment.

The fifth chapter introduces a novel approach to monitor the health of a driver while driving his car. Some vital sign measurements, as SPO2 and Heart rate, are integrated within the driving wheel and they continuously measure the cardiac activities of the driver in order to notify the health care provider and the surrounding cars in case of medical problem. The proposed system is a low cost system that aims to reduce the mortal accidents due to car crashes on road related to medical problems.

At the end, chapter six proposes both morphometric and functional connectivity analysis to investigate the underlying neural mechanisms of major depressive disorders. The analysis is based on the extraction of the cortical volume and surface area from high-resolution MRI data. As for the comparison between healthy and depressive participants, functional correlations of the structural changes were performed using a seed-based functional connectivity analysis by comparing the regions showing significant differences in the structural analysis as regions of interest (ROI).

To sum up, this book presents a general overview of the vital signs and some applications in the engineering and public health domains. Several vital sign parameter have been presented in this book along with the methods to capture, process, and analyze the resulting values.

In: Vital Signs: An Overview
Editors: Roy Abi Zeid Daou et al.
ISBN: 978-1-53617-765-7
© 2020 Nova Science Publishers, Inc.

Chapter 1

THE EFFECTS OF EXERCISE TRAINING ON BLOOD PRESSURE AMONG ADULTS

Mohammed Ali Fakhro*, DPT, Rim Fayad*
and Fatima Al Ameen
Faculty of Public Health, Department of Physical Therapy, Lebanese German University, Jounieh, Lebanon

ABSTRACT

Several large-scale epidemiology studies have clearly documented a dose-response relationship between physical activity and risk of Cardiovascular disease and premature mortality in men and women and in ethnically diverse participants. However, despite the well-documented health benefits of physical activity, physical inactivity remains a global pandemic. Therefore, in recognition of this strong link between physical activity and incidence of non-communicable diseases, member states of WHO agreed to a 10% relative reduction in the prevalence of physical inactivity by 2025, as one of the nine global targets to improve the prevention and treatment of non-communicable diseases.

---

* Corresponding Author's Email: m.fakhro@lgu.edu.lb.

Keywords: physical activity, blood pressure, intermittent exercise, continuous exercise

Despite the well-documented health benefits of physical activity (PA), physical inactivity (PI) remains a global pandemic, identified as one of the four leading contributors to premature mortality (Hallal et al., 2012; Kohl, et al, 2012). Globally, 31.1% of adults are physically inactive (Hallal et al., 2012). PI refers to people who do not meet the key age guidelines of PA (Office of Disease Prevention and Health Promotion [ODPHP], 2018).

Moreover, population-based studies have demonstrated that more than 50% of an average person's waking day involves activities associated with prolonged sitting such as television viewing and computer use (Matthews et al., 2008). This behavior is known as sedentary behavior (SB). SB is "any waking behavior characterized by an energy expenditure 1.5 or fewer minutes of moderate-intensity (METs) while sitting, reclining, or lying" (Tremblay, et al., 2017). Moreover, SB is associated with negative health consequences such as greater risk for all-cause mortality, and cardiovascular disease (CVD) (Biswas et al., 2015; Healy et al., 2008; Healy, Matthews, Dunstan, Winkler, & Owen, 2003; Katzmarzyk, Church, Craig, Bouchard, 2009; Kim, et. al., 2013), independently of PA levels (Biswas, 2015; Koster, 2012; Matthews, et al., 2012; Schwingshackl, Missbach, Dias, König, & Hoffmann, 2014). However, Data suggested that adverse outcomes associated with sedentary time decrease in magnitude among persons who are more physically active (Biswas et al., 2015).

In recognition of the strong positive correlation between PI and incidence of non-communicable diseases (NCDs), member states of WHO agreed on a 10% relative reduction in the prevalence of PI by 2025 (Target 3) (Guthold, et al., 2018). This Target is one of nine global voluntary targets with the overarching aim to reduce premature death resulting from the four major NCDs by 25% at the end of 2025 (WHO,2019). Moreover, these nine targets are created in response to the NCDs-focused target (Target 3.4) of the third health-related Sustainable Development Goals (SDG3) (WHO,2016). Target 3.4 states that by "2030 (…) one-third premature mortality from non-communicable diseases" will be reduced "through prevention and treatment and promote mental health and well-being" (WHO, 2016).

Achieving these targets is feasible through high-level political commitment, whole-of-government action and support and engagement from everyone to create the healthy environments needed to beat NCDs (WHO,2019). For that reason, the WHO made age-specific recommendations targeted at adults (18–64 yr) and older adults ($\geq$ 65 yr) as well as children and adolescents (6–17 yr) in order to reduce NCDs and other negative health conditions (WHO, 2010). Among the adults' related global recommendations for PA for health are to do at least 150 METs aerobic PA throughout the week or do at least 75 minutes of vigorous-intensity aerobic PA throughout the week or an equivalent combination of moderate- and vigorous-intensity activity. Moreover, aerobic PA should be performed in bouts of at least 10 minutes duration. For additional health benefits, adults should increase their moderate-intensity aerobic PA to 300 minutes per week, or engage in 150 minutes of vigorous-intensity aerobic physical activity per week, or an equivalent combination of both activities (WHO, 2010).

It's noteworthy that PA, exercise, and fitness are sometimes used interchangeably, and it's useful to clarify the difference between these terms. Hence, exercise is defined as "subset of PA that is planned, structured, and repetitive and has as a final or an intermediate objective the enhancement or maintenance of physical fitness" (Caspersen, et al.,1985). Exercise, like the term PA, has been often used to describe moderate-to-vigorous-intensity PA (MVPA). However, it is preferable to specify intensity when describing exercise (PAGAC, 2018). Fitness, on the other hand, is defined as "the ability to carry out daily tasks with vigor and alertness, without undue fatigue, and with ample energy to enjoy leisure-time pursuits and respond to emergencies" (Centers for Disease Control and Prevention [CDC], 2018), others stratify physical fitness into health- or skill-related attributes (Caspersen, et al.,1985).

In order to reduce the economic burden associated with PI, along with enhancing quality of life, effective strategies to promote adequate and consistent engagement in PA are needed especially for the time-limited worker. Therefore, the 2018 Physical Activity Guidelines for Americans, recommended that PA be accumulated in bouts of at least 10 minutes in duration to influence a variety of health-related outcomes. However, additional evidence, mostly from cross-sectional studies, suggests that PA accumulated in bouts that are less than 10 minutes is also associated with favorable health-related outcomes.

Evidence to support the inverse relationship between regular PA and/or exercise and premature mortality, CVD/coronary artery disease (CAD), hypertension and a lot of other negative health conditions continues to accumulate (Garber, et al., 2011; Moore, et al., 2016; Physical Activity Guidelines Advisory Committee [PAGAC], 2018). Several large-scale epidemiology studies have clearly documented a dose-response relationship between PA and risk of CVD and premature mortality in men and women and in ethnically diverse participants (Lee, Rexrode, Cook, Manson, & Buring, 2001; Manson, et al., 2002; Naci,& Ioannidis, 2013; Paffenbarger, et., al., 1993; PAGAC, 2008; Tanasescu, et al., 2002; Yu, Yarnell, Sweetnam, Murray, 2003). It is also important to note that aerobic capacity (i.e., CRF) has an inverse relationship with risk of premature death from all causes and specifically from CVD, and higher levels of CRF are associated with higher levels of habitual PA, which in turn are associated with many health benefits (Blair, et al., 1989; Blair, et al., 1995; Garber, et al., 2011; Kodama, et al., 2009; Sesso, Paffenbarger, & Lee, 2000; Wang, et al., 2010; Williams, 2001; Williams, 2013). PA is defined as "any bodily movement produced by skeletal muscles that result in energy expenditure" (Caspersen et al., 1985).

More specifically, exercise is considered an important health behavior for the primary prevention and treatment of hypertension, which remains a common and important risk factor for cardiovascular and renal diseases (Hegde, & Solomon, 2015). Exercise is associated with an immediate significant decrease in systolic blood pressure (SBP) that can persist for almost 24 hours after exercise (Pescatello, et al., 2004). This is referred to as post-exercise hypotension, and the most pronounced effects were seen in those with higher baseline blood pressure (BP) (Pescatello, et al., 2004). Moreover, a cohort study demonstrated that PA in bouts of either at least

10 minutes or less than 10 minutes in duration was associated with lower incidence of hypertension (White, Gabriel, Kim, Lewis, & Sternfeld, 2015). Two other cross-sectional studies showed that PA accumulated in bouts less than 10 minutes was associated with lower resting BP (Loprinzi, & Cardinal, 2013; Wolff-Hughes, Fitzhugh, Bassett, Churilla, 2015). The decrease in BP after PA is thought to be due to reduction in peripheral vascular resistance (Harmer, 2006). Other proposed mechanisms for blood pressure reduction include favorable changes in oxidative stress, inflammation, endothelial function, arterial compliance, body mass, renin-angiotensin system activity, parasympathetic activity, renal function, and insulin sensitivity (Diaz, & Shimbo, 2013).

The intermittent exercise involves short frequent bouts of activity, spread throughout the day. Intermittent or fractionized exercise has emerged as a novel alternative of long bouts of exercise, since it showed similar effect in eliciting post-exercise hypotension and maximizing blood pressure control throughout the day (Angadi, S. S., Weltman, A., Watson-Winfield, D., Weltman, J., Frick, K., Patrie, J., & Gaesser, G. A.,2010). Moreover, many studies have demonstrated the acute effects that of 67 intermittent exercise on lowering BP (Angadi et al., 2010; Bhammar et al., 2012; Jones, Taylor et al., 2009; Miyashita, Burns, & Stensel, 2011; Miyashita et al., 2008; Padilla, Wallace, & Park, 2005; Park, Rink, & Wallace, 2008; Park, Rink, & Wallace, 2006; Taylor-Tolbert et al., 2000). Moreover, Bhammar et al., 2012 showed that 10-min of intermittent aerobic exercise performed three times/day, was effective in reducing 24 h SBP. They also showed that intermittent exercise was more effective in significantly reducing nighttime SBP and in attenuating the early morning rise in SBP as compared to continuous exercise. Intermittent exercise is also effective in increasing cardiovascular fitness (Debusk, Stenestrand, Sheehan, & Haskell, 1990; Donnelly, Jacobsen, Heelan, Seip, & Smith, 2000), decreasing lipemia (Altena, Michaelson, Ball, & Thomas, 2004) and arterial stiffness (Tordi, Mourot, Colin, & Regnard, 2010).

The 2018 Physical Activity Guidelines for Americans, showed that aerobic intermittent training performed twice a day had similar effects as continuous aerobic training on a variety of CVD risk factors. These effects include an improvement in the status of metabolic syndrome, a decrease in C-reactive protein, a decrease in high-density lipoprotein, reduction of waist circumference, and a decrease in subcutaneous fat as measured by triceps and subscapular skinfold measurements (Schmidt, Biwer, & Kalscheuer, 2001).

Given that a lack of time is a frequently cited barrier to physical activity, intermittent exercise is considered easier, and more feasible than continuous aerobic exercise, especially by employees who lack time for daily exercise. Moreover, intermittent exercise decreases the burden associated with PI and enhances an active lifestyle (Eguchi, Ohta & Yamato, 2013; Trost, Owen, Bauman, Sallis, Brown, 2001).

These findings are of public health importance because it suggests that engaging in PA, regardless of the length of the bout, may have health-enhancing effects. This is of particular importance for individuals who are unwilling or unable to engage in physical activity bouts that are at least 10 minutes in duration. Therefore, public health initiatives to enhance health should recommend including PA as an important lifestyle behavior regardless of the duration.

REFERENCES

Angadi, SS, A Weltman, D Watson-Winfield, J. Weltman, K Frick, J Patrie, and G A Gaesser. "Effect of fractionized vs continuous, single-session exercise on blood pressure in adults." *Journal of Human Hypertension* 24, no.4 (2010): 300-302. doi:10.1038/jhh.2009.110.

Bhammar, Dharini, Siddhartha Angadi, and Glenn Gasser." Effects of fractionized and continuous exercise on 24-h ambulatory blood pressure." *Medicine and Science in Sports and Exercise* 44, no.12(2012):2270–2276. doi:10.1249/MSS.0b013e3182663117.

Biswas, Aviroop, Paul I. Oh, Guy E. Faulkner, Ravi R. Bajaj, Michael A. Silver, Marc S. Mitchell, and David A. Alter. "Sedentary time and its association with risk for disease incidence, mortality, and hospitalization in adults: a systematic review and meta-analysis." *Ann. Intern. Med.* 162, no. 2 (2015):123–32. doi:10.736/m14-1651.

Blair, Steven N, Harold W. Kohl, Ralph S. Paffenbarger Jr. Debra G. Clark, Kenneth H. Cooper, Larry W. Gibbons." Physical fitness and all-cause mortality. A prospective study of healthy men and women." *JAMA* 262, no.17(1989): 2395–401.doi:10.1001/jama.1989.03430170057028.

Blair, Steven N., Harold W. Kohl, Carolyn E. Barlow, Ralph S., Paffenbarger, Larry W. Gibbons, and Carol Macera. "Changes in physical fitness and all-cause mortality. A prospective study of healthy and unhealthy men." *JAMA* 273, no.14 (1995):1093–8. doi:10.1001/jama.1995.03520380029031.

Caspersen, Carl J., Kenneth E. Powell, Gregory M. Christenson. "Physical Activity, Exercise, and Physical Fitness: Definitions and Distinctions for Health-Related Research." *Public Health Reports* 100, no.2 (1985). Stable URL: http://www.jstor.org/stable/20056429 (Accessed: 04-01-2016 08:39 UTC).

Centers for Disease Control and Prevention. Physical fitness. In CDC Glossary of Terms.

DeBusk, Robert F., Ulf Stenestrand, Mary Sheehan, and William L. Haskell. "Training effects of long versus short bouts of exercise in healthy subjects." *American Journal of Cardiology* 65, no.15 (1990): 1010-1013.DOI:https://doi.org/10.1016/0002-9149(90)91005-Q.

Diaz, Keith M., and Daichi Shimbo. "Physical activity and the prevention of hypertension." *Current hypertension reports* 15, no 6(2013): 659–668.doi:10.1007/s11906-013-0386-8.

Eguch, Masafumi, Masanori, and Hiroshi Yamato." The effects of single long and accumulated short bouts of exercise on cardiovascular risks in male Japanese workers: a randomized controlled study." *Industrial health*, 51, no. 6 (2013): 563–571.doi:10.2486/indhealth.2013-0023.

Garber, Carole E., Michael R Deschenes, Michael J. Lamonte, David Christopher Nieman, Bryan Blissmer, Bryan Blissmer, I-Min Lee, and David P Swain ."American College of Sports Medicine position stand. The quantity and quality of exercise for developing and maintaining cardiorespiratory, musculoskeletal, and neuromotor fitness in apparently healthy adults: guidance for prescribing exercise." *Med. Sci. Sports Exerc.* 43, no. 7 (2011):1334–559. doi:10.1249/mss.0b013e3 182 13fefb.

Guthold, Regina, Gretchen A Stevens, Leanne M Riley, and Prof Fiona C Bull. "Worldwide trends in insufficient physical activity from 2001 to 2016: A pooled analysis of 358 population-based surveys with 1·9 million participants." *The Lancet Global Health* 6, no. 10 (2018):e1077–e1086. doi.org/10.1016/S2214-109X(18)30357-7.

Hallal, Pedro C., Lars Bo Andersen, Fiona C Bull, Regina Guthold and William Haskell." *Global physical activity levels: surveillance progress, pitfalls, and prospects." The Lancet* 380, no .9838 (2012): 247–257. doi: 10.1016/s0140-6736(12)60646-1.

Hamer, Mark, Adrian Taylor, Andrew Steptoe Taylor. "The effect of acute aerobic exercise on stress-related blood pressure response: a systematic review and meta-analysis." *Biol. Psycho.* 71, no. 2 (2006): 183-90. DOI:10.1016/j.biopsycho.2005.04.004.

Healy, Genevieve N., Charles E. Matthews, David W. Dunstan, Elisabeth A.H. Winkler, and Neville Owen. "Sedentary time and cardio-metabolic biomarkers in US adults: NHANES 2003-06," *Eur. Heart J.* 32, no. 5 (2011):590–7. doi.org/10.1093/eurheartj/ehq451.

Healy, Genevieve N., David W. Dunstan, Jo Salmon, Ester Cerin, Jonathan E. Shaw, Paul Z. Zimmet, and Neville Owen. "Breaks in Sedentary Time: Beneficial associations with metabolic risk," *Diabetes Care 31, no. 4* (2008)*: 661–666.* doi: 10.2337/dc07-2046.

Hegde, Sheila M., Scott D. Solomon. "Influence of Physical Activity on Hypertension and Cardiac Structure and Function," *Current hypertension reports* 17, no .10 (2015): 77. doi:10.1007/s11906-015-05883. http://www.health.gov/paguidelines/Report/pdf/Committee Report.pdf.https://www.cdc.gov/physicalactivity/basics/glossary/index. htm. (*Accessed January*, 30, 2018). https://www.cdc. gov/physical activity/basics/glossary/index.htm. (Accessed January 30, 2018).

JE, Donnelly, Jacobsen DJ, Heelan KS, Seip R, and Smith S. "The effects of 18 months of intermittent vs continuous exercise on aerobic capacity, body weight and composition and metabolic fitness in previously sedentary, moderately obese females." *International Journal of Obesity* 24, no. 5 (2000): 566–572.doi: 10.1038/sj.ijo.0801198.

Jones, Helen, Chloe E. Taylor, Nia C. S. Lewis, Keith George, and Greg Atkinson. "Post-exercise blood pressure reduction is greater following intermittent than continuous exercise and is influenced less by diurnal variation," *Chronobiology International* 26, no. 2(2009):293-306. doi: 10.1080/07420520902739717.

Katzmarzyk, Peter, Timothy Church, Cora Craig, and Claude Bouchard. "Sitting time and mortality from all causes, cardiovascular disease, and cancer," *Med. Sci. Sports Exerc.* 41, no. 5(2009):998–1005. DOI: 10.1249/MSS.0b013e3181930355.

Kim, Yeonju, Lynne R Wilkens, Song-Yi Park, Marc T Goodman, Kristine R Monroe, and Laurence N Kolonel. "Association between various sedentary behaviours and all-cause, cardiovascular disease and cancer mortality: the Multiethnic Cohort Study." *Int. J. Epidemiol.* 42, no.4(2013):1040–56. doi.org/10.1093/ije/dyt108.

Kodama, Satoru, Shiro Tanaka, Miho Maki, Yoko Yachi, Mihoko Asumi, Ayumi Sugawara, and Kumiko Totsuka, et al. "Cardiorespiratory fitness as a quantitative predictor of all-cause mortality and cardiovascular events in healthy men and women: a meta-analysis." *JAMA* 301, no. 19(2009):2024–35, doi:10.1001/jama.2009.681.

Kohl, Harold W, Cora Lynn Craig, Estelle Victoria Lambert, Shigeru Inoue, Jasem Ramadan Alkandari, Grit Leetongin, and Sonja Kahlmeier."The pandemic of physical inactivity: global action for public health." *The Lancet 380, no. 9838* (2012): *294–305.* doi: 10.1016/s0140-6736(12)60898-8.

Koster, Annemarie, Paolo Caserotti, Kushang V. Patel, Charles E. Matthews, David Berrigan, Dane R. Van Domelen, Robert J. Brychta, Kong Y. Chen, and Tamara B. Harris. "Association of Sedentary Time with Mortality Independent of Moderate to Vigorous Physical Activity." *PLoS ONE* 7, no.6(2012): *e37696*.doi:10.1371/journal.pone.0037696 .

Lee, Min, Kathryn M. Rexrode, Nancy R. Cook, JoAnn E. Manson, and Julie E. Buring. "Physical activity and coronary heart disease in women: is "no pain, no gain" passe?" *JAMA* 285, no. 11(2001):1447–54. doi:10.1001/jama.285.11.1447.

Loprinzi, Paul D., and Bradley J. Cardinal." Association between biologic outcomes and objectively measured physical activity accumulated in >/=10-minute bouts and < 10-minute bouts." *Am J Health Promot* 27, no. 3(2013):143–151. doi:10.4278/ajhp.110916-QUAN-348.

Manson, JoAnn E., Philip Greenland, Andrea Z. LaCroix, Marcia L. Stefanick, Charles P. Mouton, Albert Oberman, Michael G. Perri, et al. "Walking compared with vigorous exercise for the prevention of cardiovascular events in women," *N. Engl. J. Med.* 347, no.10 (2002):716–25. DOI: 10.1056/NEJMoa021067.

Matthews, Charles E., Stephanie M George, Steven C Moore, Heather R Bowles, Aaron Blair, Yikyung Park, Richard P Troiano, Albert Hollenbeck, and Arthur Schatzkin. "Amount of time spent in sedentary behaviors and cause-specific mortality in US adults." *Am. J. Clin. Nutr.* 95, no.2 (2012): 437–45. doi.org/10.3945/ajcn.111.019620.

Matthews, Charles E., Kong Y. Chen, Patty S. Freedson, Maciej S. Buchowski, Bettina M. Beech, Russell R. Pate, and Richard P. Troiano." Amount of time spent in sedentary behaviors in the United States, 2003–2004." *Am. J. Epidemiol.* 167, no. 7(2008):875–81. doi.org/10.1093/aje/kwm390.

Miyashita, Masashi, Stephen F. Burns, and David J. Stensel. "Accumulating short bouts of running reduces resting blood pressure in young normotensive/pre-hypertensive men." *Journal of Sports Sciences* 29, no.14 (2011): 1473-1482. doi:10.1080/02640414.2011.593042.

Miyashita, Masashi, Stephen F. Burns, and David J. Stensel." Accumulating short bouts of brisk walking reduces postprandial plasma triacylglycerol concentrations and resting blood pressure in healthy young men." *American Journal of Clinical Nutrition* 88, no. 5 (2008):1225-1231.doi:10.3945/ajcn.2008.26493.

Moore, teven C., I-Min Lee, Elisabete Weiderpass, Peter T. Campbell, Joshua N. Sampson, Cari M. Kitahara, Sarah K. KeadleSC, Lee I, Weiderpass E, et al. "Association of leisure-time physical activity with risk of 26 types of cancer in 1.44 million adults." *JAMA Intern Med* 176, no. 6 (2016):816–25: doi:10.1001 jama intern med.2016.1548.

Naci, Huseyin, and John P A Ioannidis. "Comparative effectiveness of exercise and drug interventions on mortality outcomes: meta-epidemiological study," *BMJ* 347, no.5 (2013): 347:f5577. https://doi.org/10.1136/bmj.f5577 (accessed 01 October 2013).

Office of Disease Prevention and Health Promotion. *PA Guidelines Advisory Committee submitted its Scientific Repor,* (2018). *t.* Retrieved from https://health.gov/paguidelines/second-edition/report/?

Padilla, Jaume, Janet Wallace, and Sejong Park." Accumulation of physical activity reduces blood pressure in pre- and hypertension." *Medicine and Science in Sports and Exercise* 37, no. 8(2005): 1264-1275,doi:10.1249/01.mss.0000175079.23850.95.

Paffenbarger, Ralph S., Robert T. Hyde, Alvin L. Wing, I-Min Lee, Dexter L. Jung, and James B. Kampert. "The association of changes in physical-activity level and other lifestyle characteristics with mortality among men." *N. Engl. J. Med.* 328, no. 8(1993):538–45. DOI: 10.1056/NEJM199302253280804.

Park, S, LD Rink, and JP Wallace. "Accumulation of physical activity: Blood pressure reduction between 10-min walking sessions." *Journal of Human Hypertension* 22, no. 7(2008): 475-482, doi:10.1038/jhh.2008.29.

Park, Saejon, Lawrence Rink, and Janet Wallace." Accumulation of physical activity leads to a greater blood pressure reduction than a single continuous session, in prehypertension," *Journal of Hypertension* 24, no. 9(2006): 1761-1770. DOI: 10.1097/01.hjh.0000242400.37967.54.

Pate, Russell R., Michael Pratt, Steven N. Blair, William L. Haskell, Caroline A. Macera, Claude Bouchard, David Buchner, et al., "Physical-activity and public-health-a recommendation from the Centers-for disease-Control-and-Prevention and the American-

College-of-Sports-Medicin." *JAMA* 273, no. 5(1995): 402-7. doi:10.1001/jama.1995.03520290054029.

Pescatello, Linda, Barry Franklin, Robert Fagard, William Farquhar, George Kelley, and Chester Ray." American College of Sports Medicine." *Med. Sci. Sports Exerc.* 36, no. 3(2004):533-53. DOI: 10.1249/01.MSS.0000115224.88514.3A.

Schmidt, Dan, Craig J. Biwer, and Linda K. Kalscheuer" Effects of long versus short bout exercise on fitness and weight loss in overweight female." *J. Am. CollNutr.* 20, no.5 (2001):494-501. DOI: 10.1080/07315724.2001.10719058.

Schwingshackl, Lukas, Benjamin Missbach, Sofia Dias, Jürgen König, and Georg Hoffmann." Impact of different training modalities on glycaemic control and blood lipids in patients with type 2 diabetes: a systematic review and network meta-analysis," *Diabetologia* 57, no.9(2014).):1789–97. doi:10.1007/s00125-014-3303-z.

Sesso, Howard D., Ralph S. PaffenbargerJr, and I-Min Lee." Physical activity and coronary heart disease in men: the Harvard Alumni Health Study."*Circulation* 102, no.9 (2000).):975–80.d oi.org/10.1161/01.CIR.102.9.975.

Tanasescu, Mihaela, Michael F. Leitzmann, Eric B. Rimm, Walter C. Willett, Meir J. Stampfer, and Frank B. Hu." Exercise type and intensity in relation to coronary heart disease in men." *JAMA* 288, no.16 (2002):1994–2000. doi:10.1001/jama.288.16.1994.

Taylor-Tolbert, Nadine S., Donald R. Dengel, Michael D. Brown, Steve D. McCole, Richard E. Pratley, Robert E. Ferrell, and James M. Hagberg. "Ambulatory blood pressure after acute exercise in older men with essential hypertension." *Am. J. Hypertens* 13, no. 1(2000).): 44-51. doi.org/10.1016/S0895-7061(99)00141-7.

Tomas, Altena, Jody Michaelson, Steven ball and Tom Thomas. "Single sessions of intermittent and continuous exercise and postprandial lipemia."*Medicine and Science in Sports and Exercise* 36, no.8 (2004):1364-1371. doi:10.1249/MSS.0000135793.43808.6C.

Tordi, Nicolas, Laurent Mourot, Eglantine Colin, and Jacques Regnard." Intermittent versus constant aerobic exercise: Effects on arterial stiffness." *European Journal of Applied Physiology* 108, no. 4(2010): 801-809, doi:10.1007/s00421-009-1285-1.

Tremblay, Mark S., Salomé Aubert, Joel D. Barnes, Travis J. Saunders,Valerie Carson, Amy E. Latimer-Cheung, Sebastien F.M. Chastin, et al. "Sedentary Behavior Research Network (SBRN) – Terminology Consensus Project process and outcome." *In.t J. Behav. Nutr. Phys. Act* .14, no.75(2017): doi:10.1186/s12966-017-0525-8.

Trost, Stewart G., Neville Owen, Adrian E. Bauman, James F. Sallis, and Wendy Brown." Correlates of adults' participation in physical activity: review and update." *Med. Sci. Sports Exerc.* 34, no. 12 (2001): 1996-2001. doi:10.1097/00005768-200212000-00020.

Wang, Chia-Yih, William L. Haskell, Stephen W. Farrell, Michael J. LaMonte, Steven N. Blair, Lester R. Curtin, Jeffery P. Hughes, and Vicki L. Burt." Cardiorespiratory fitness levels among US adults 20-49 years of age: findings from the 1999-2004 National Health and Nutrition Examination Survey." *Am. J. Epidemiol.* 17, no. 4(2010):426–35. doi.org/10.1093/aje/kwp412.

White, Daniel, Kelley Gabriel, Yongin Kim, Cora Lewis, and Barbara Sternefd." Do Short Spurts of Physical Activity Benefit Cardiovascular Health? The CARDIA Study." *Medicine and science in sports and exercise* 47, no. 11(2015):2353–2358. doi:10.1249/MSS.000000 000 0000662.

WHO, Physical Activity and Adults. (2019). *Who.int.* Retrieved 15 November 2019, from https://www.who.int/dietphysicalactivity/ factsheet_adults/en/.

Williams, Paul T." Dose-response relationship of physical activity to premature and total all-cause and cardiovascular disease mortality in walkers," *PLoS One* 8, no. 11 (2013): e78777.DOI:10.1371/ journal.pone.0078777.

Williams, Paul T." Physical fitness and activity as separate heart disease risk factors: a meta-analysis." *Med. Sci. Sports Exerc.* 33, no.5 (2001):754–61.DOI:10.1097/00005768-200105000-00012.

Wolff-Hughes, Dana L., Eugene C. Fitzhugh, David R.Bassett, and James R. Churilla. "Total activity counts and bouted minutes of moderate-to-vigorous physical activity: relationships with cardiometabolic biomarkers using 2003–2006NHANES." *J. Phys. Act Health,* 12, no. 5 (2015): 694–700. doi:10.1123/jpah.2013-0463.

Yu, S, J W G Yarnell, P M Sweetnam, L Murray" What level of physical activity protects against premature cardiovascular death?" *The Caerphilly study Heart* 89, no. 5 (2003):502–6. http://dx.doi.org/10.1136/heart.89.5.502.

In: Vital Signs: An Overview
Editors: Roy Abi Zeid Daou et al.
ISBN: 978-1-53617-765-7
© 2020 Nova Science Publishers, Inc.

Chapter 2

THE EFFECT OF SURGICAL STRESS ON VITAL SIGNS AND NURSING CARE

Selda Mert Boğa[1] and Aylin Aydin Sayilan[2]
[1]PhD, Kocaeli Vocational School of Health Services, Kocaeli University, Kocaeli, Turkey
[2]Assist. Prof. Dr. Kırklareli University Department of Nursing, Kırklareli, Turkey

ABSTRACT

Although surgical procedures can be life-saving, the decision to operate inevitably causes stress in patients. That stress results in physiological and psychological responses. Neuro-endocrine responses occur while waiting in the preoperative period. These can then result in physiological changes in vital signs, including elevated heart and respiratory rates and blood pressure, and pain. It is therefore essential to ensure that the patient is physiologically and psychologically prepared in the preoperative period. The patient's ability to cope with potential problems relies on good preparation and support. By providing appropriate care before, during and after surgery, the nurse should manage care while ensuring patients are able to cope with the trauma of the operation and potential complications.

Keywords: surgical stress, vital signs, nursing care

INTRODUCTION

Admission to hospital for surgery can create stress in many individuals. Waiting for surgery can result in a neuro-endocrine response in the preoperative period. Physiologically, changes are seen in vital signs such as increased heart and respiratory rates, and blood pressure elevation. Psychologically, signs and symptoms of lack of appetite and lethargy may be seen. Providing psychological support is a basic nursing task in reducing stress before surgery, while regular monitoring of vital signs is a basic nursing procedure in preventing postoperative complications.

1. THE DEVELOPMENT OF STRESS REACTIONS TO SURGICAL PROCEDURES

Stress is defined as the body's reaction to stressors. Hans Selye refers to a general adaptation syndrome whereby the body may react to stressors with a local response at the cellular and tissue level, or with a systemic response causing changes in blood pressure, heart rate, body temperature, and fluid-electrolyte balance. When the organism encounters a powerful stressor such as surgery, the hypothalamus is stimulated. This affects the sympathetic nervous system (SNS) and pituitary gland, and various hormones are then released. Epinephrine and norepinephrine are secreted from the medulla of the adrenal gland with stimulation of the SNS as a result of a neuro-endocrine response to pain. Under the effect of epinephrine, heart rate and myocardial contractility increase, which in turn increases the workload of the heart and myocardial O2 (Siedlecki 2009; Smeltzer et al., 2010; Ledowski et al., 2012; Renn & Leslie 2012; Adib Hajbaghery at al., 2014; Younessi Heravi et al., 2015). Blood pressure increases as a result of constriction caused by norepinephrine in peripheral vessels, and a pale appearance emerges as the skin cools. In addition, superficial vasoconstriction can lead to venous stasis and blood clotting (thromboembolic complications) by resulting in reduced blood flow. Bronchodilation and a rapid increase in respiration rate (rapid and superficial respiration) are observed with stimulation of the respiration center in the medulla. Adrenocorticotropic hormone (ACTH) is released from the anterior pituitary and antidiuretic hormone (ADH) from the posterior pituitary as a result of the effect of the hypothalamus on the pituitary. ACTH causes the release of aldosterone and glucocorticoid by affecting the adrenal gland cortex. Aldosterone leads to reabsorption of sodium, and thus of water, from the kidney, as a result of which blood volume increases, urine levels decrease (due to hypermotility of the urethra and bladder), and blood pressure also increases. This leads to the release of ADH from the posterior pituitary. Glucocorticoids increase blood glucose levels by converting protein and fats into glucose (Erdil and Özhan Elbaş 2008; Siedlecki 2009; Smeltzer et al., 2010; Ledowski et al., 2012; Renn & Leslie 2012) (Figure 1).

The stress reaction protects the body against surgical trauma. Preservation of homeostatic balance broadly depends on the effectiveness of the stress reaction, which is itself dependent on the age and physiological and psychological condition of the individual scheduled for surgery, and the duration of the stress.

2. VITAL SIGNS AND NURSING CARE IN THE PERIOPERATIVE PERIOD

The term 'perioperative' comprises the preoperative (before surgery), intraoperative (during surgery), and postoperative (after surgery) stages. Each phase involves a specific time in th surgical experience, and each requires a variety of specific nursing behaviors and procedures. The aim of perioperative nursing is to provide perfect patient care before, during, and after surgery. Nursing activities are intended to meet the patient's urgent physical and psychosocial needs. Every patient has different expectation regarding the surgical experience and different hopes concerning outcomes of surgery. The nurse plays an active role in the entire perioperative period to ensure the quality and continuity of patient care (White et al., 2013).

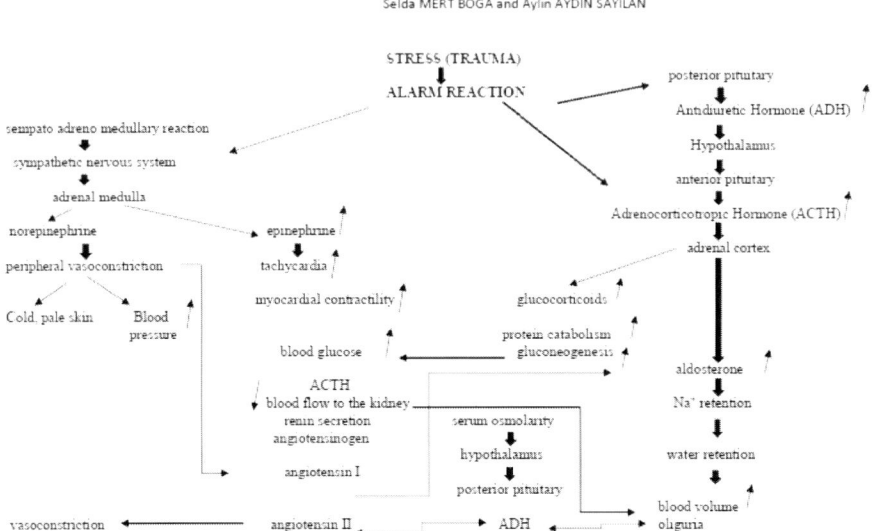

Erdil, F and Özhan Elbaş, N. *Cerrahi Hastalıkları Hemşireliği*. 5th ed. Ankara, Aydoğdu Ofset, 2008, 123-136.

Figure 1. The body's neuro-endocrine reaction to stress.

2.1. Preoperative Phase

The preoperative phase with the patient's decision to undergo surgery, and ends with the patient being placed on the operating table. Even if very well planned beforehand, surgery is nevertheless a stressor that produces both psychological (anxiety and fear) and physiological (neuroendocrine) stress reactions. The surgical patient is at risk in terms of the procedure and the operative outcome. The patient is evaluated psychologically and physiologically by the nurse during this phase.

Patient psychological well-being has an effect on the operative outcome. Fear and anxiety are normal reactions to surgical stress and affect the patient's ability to cope with the recommended care plan. Since patients' perceptions of the significance of surgery vary, the degree of fear and anxiety is also variable. In case of excessive fear and anxiety, these emotions can hinder healing by magnifying the normal physiological stress reaction. The nurse can provide support and information by evaluating the patient's fears and anxieties. Fear of the unknown (pain, disability, anesthesia, fear of death, etc.) is the most widespread preoperative fear. However, this fear can be easily overcome by the burse by means of patient education and preoperative instruction (providing information concerning such areas as premedication, the length of the surgical procedure, special skin preparation, incision type, and the postoperative care unit).

Preoperative education commences the moment the patient agrees to surgery. Information provided by phone or e-mailed before surgery can be highly beneficial. Immediately prior to surgery, a brief review of preoperative education is performed with additional information specific to the individual patient's requirements. The patient must always be given the opportunity to ask questions. Information must always be tailored to the patient's requirements and knowledge and anxiety levels. Mild to moderate anxiety is a positive factor that increases alertness and acts as an encouragement to learning. Mildly anxious patients will be given the most comprehensive instructions. Moderately anxious patients are given less information, but this is more directed toward specific subjects of concern. Very anxious patients are given only elementary information, but they are also encouraged to raise any concerns they may have. Patients in a state of panic cannot learn anything. No information is provided in such cases, but the surgeon is notified accordingly.

Changes in physiological functions are reflected in vital sign values. Deviations from normal values show that homeostasis is impaired or interrupted (Oktay et al., 2017). Vital signs must be assessed at specific intervals in order to evaluate an individual's physiological functions. The frequency at which vital signs are evaluated depends on the patient's state of health, the procedures being performed, and the physician's instructions. Assessment, measurement and monitoring of vital signs is an important and basic cursing skill. Before the surgical procedure, the nurse must check such vital signs as blood pressure, temperature, pulse, and respiration. The presence of some anxiety-induced changes in vital signs is normal. However, the surgeon must be informed in case of marked variations in basic data (White et al., 2013).

2.2. Intraoperative Phase

The intraoperative phase refers to the time elapsing during surgery, beginning with the patient being placed on the operating table and ending with admission to the post-anesthesia care unit (PACU).

Oxygenation and Ventilation

Almost all anesthetics are respiratory depressants. Benzodiazepines, opioids, and inhalation anesthetic agents exhibit a significant depressive effect on respiration. Any of these drugs can cause apnea (cessation of airflow exceeding 10 sec) during general anesthesia. When employed together, their impact on respiration is combinative. When the rate or depth of respiration is reduced, carbon dioxide elimination is delayed, and carbon dioxide accumulates in the blood and lungs. Oxygen saturation is observed using a pulse oximeter. Even a small amount of additional oxygen administered to a patient with reduced bleeding time or respiration depth makes a significant contribution to the amount of oxygen in the blood stream. This explains why oxygen is even administered to healthy patients during recovery from general anesthesia (White et al., 2013).

Heart Rate and Blood Pressure

Few direct changes in heart rate and blood pressure regulation occur in patients recovering from general anesthesia. Some largely opioid-based anesthetic techniques, including fentanyl citrate (Sublimaze) or sufentanil citrate (Sufenta), can result in a slow heart rate, although no specific action is required as long as blood pressure is maintained. Although most general anesthetics are myocardial depressants, the depressive effects of today's agents are mild, particularly once anesthetic administration has been terminated.

The majority of changes in heart rate and blood pressure during recovery are due to factors indirectly associated with the anesthetic. Heart rate and blood pressure both rise as a result of sympathetic stimulation. Pain, hypoxia, and fear give rise to sympathetic stimulation and a resulting increase in heart rate and blood pressure. Identifying and addressing the source of patient fear frequently lowers anxiety levels. Heart rate and blood pressure may both be expected to return to normal when the factors responsible for sympathetic stimulation are addressed (White et al., 2013).

Temperature Regulation and Shivering

Under general anesthesia, the body's natural thermoregulation capacity is lost. General anesthetics expand the superficial blood vessels. This results in warm blood being exposed to the cooler exterior. During anesthetization, the patient is in a cold operating room in an uncovered state, and cold solutions are applied in order to cleanse the operative site. When the surgical procedure commences, the patient's insulation layers (skin and subcutaneous fat) are opened to reveal the warm interior of the body and allow heat to escape. In addition, intravenous (IV) fluids at room temperature are infused into the veins, and the patient inhales cool gases. Surgical patients lose considerable quantities of heat just when the body is least capable of warming the tissues. Hypothermia exacerbates depression of the central nervous system (CNS) caused by any remaining anesthetics. One effective means of increasing body temperature intraoperatively and during recovery from general anesthesia is by means of surface warming with a forced-air warming blanket. Warm cloth blankets also conserve body warmth.

Shivering is observed with all potent inhalation agents during emergence from general anesthesia, a time when blood levels of anesthetic agents are very low. The reason for this shivering is not yet fully understood, but seems to be independent of the patient's body temperature. Shivering is of course also observed in postoperative patients when they are cold. Postoperative shivering can be eliminated by keeping the patient warm and by encouraging deep breathing to facilitate rapid elimination of the anesthetic agent (White et al., 2013).

2.3. Postoperative Phase

The postoperative phase commences with the completion of the surgical procedure and until discharge, from the hospital or institution, but also from medical care by the operating surgeon.

Postoperative Nursing Care

The post-anesthesia nurse records the patient's time of arrival at the unit and immediately evaluates airway patency by placing a hand above the subject's face to assess exhalation. The quality and quantity of respirations are then observed, together with the presence of an artificial airway. The patient is attached to a pulse oximeter, and respiratory sounds are auscultated. The nurse also observes the color and condition of the skin as another component of respiratory evaluation. Presence of circumoral pallor is also checked from the lips. Peripheral cyanosis may be suggestive of hypothermia, rather than of respiratory distress (White et al., 2013).

Continuing Nursing Care in the PACU

The post-anesthesia nurse employs a separate nursing record for the PACU. It is highly important for any unusual events to be fully recorded. If vital signs are within normal limits, the post-anesthesia nurse checks these every 15 minutes. In case of unstable vital signs, these are monitored every 5 minutes or as required until stability is achieved. The surgeon and anesthesia provider must be informed if vital signs fail to normalize. The surgical site is checked a minimum of once every 30 minutes. The surgeon must be informed if any initial bleeding fails to subside. Routine checks are maintained until discharge from the PACU.

The post-anesthesia nurse determines whether the patient meets the criteria for discharge from the PACU. This is generally when vital signs are stable and within the patient's normal limits (White et al., 2013).

Later Postoperative Nursing Care

When the patient arrives at the clinical unit, the nurse assists in putting the patient to bed. A brief evaluation, including vital signs, is conducted every 15 minutes for 1 hour, every 30 minutes for 2 hours, and every hour for 4 hours, or as requested by the physician.

Post-anesthetic complications may still occur during this time, although these differ as time passes. The nurse is responsible for their management:

1. *Ineffective airway clearance* may develop due to atelectasis and hypostatic pneumonia. Respiratory complications be seen in any anesthetized patient. As in the PACU, patients are at risk of ineffective airway clearance, ineffective breathing patterns, and aspiration during the postoperative period. However, contemporary nursing procedures are aimed at preventing ineffective airway clearance caused by atelectasis and hypostatic pneumonia, both of which usually occur within the first 48 hours postoperatively. Postoperative atelectasis involves the pulmonary bronchioles becoming clogged by mucus, effectively preventing air from reaching the alveoli, which then collapse. Dyspnea, fever, tachypnea, tachycardia, and cyanosis may develop. Postoperative hypostatic pneumonia is a condition in which stagnant mucus facilitates bacterial growth, with atelectasis subsequently developing into a secondary infection.

It is important to actively encourage the patient to cough, breathe deeply (with and without incentive spirometry), and to turn as instructed preoperatively if these sequelae are to be avoided. The patient must also be motivated to sit up and walk as early and frequently as instructed. Analgesia must also be ensured so that mobility is well tolerated (White et al., 2013).

2. The patient may also become at risk for *disturbed sensory perception* associated with anesthesia, narcotics, change of environment, fluid and electrolyte imbalances, sleep deprivation, hypoxia, and sensory deprivation or overload. *Hypothermia* may be seen in association with anesthesia and the surgical environment, or *hyperthermia* in the presence

of infection. Neurological function disturbance may vary and manifest in the form of pain, fever, or delirium.

Hypothermia is frequently seen in the first few hours postoperatively. Blankets should be offered as required. Due to the normal inflammatory response occurring, body temperature may subsequently increase to a low-level fever. The surgeon must be informed if the patient's body temperature exceeds 38°C. Atelectasis and dehydration result in temperature elevation (exceeding 38°C) in the first 24 to 48 hours postoperatively. If body temperature still exceeds 38°C 48 hours after surgery, then a wound, respiratory or urinary tract infection, thrombophlebitis, or pulmonary embolism should be suspected.

The nurse's primary function is to obviate infection by means of proper aseptic technique. In case of fever, the cause of the elevation must be ascertained through the collection of urine, wound, blood, or sputum cultures. Antipyretics must be administered as instructed. Patient comfort can be enhanced by providing light covers and clothing, frequent linen changes, cool flannels, and maintaining a cool environment (White et al., 2013).

REFERENCES

Adib, Hajbaghery, M., Moradi, T. and Mohseni, R, "Effects of a multimodal preparation package on vital signs of patients waiting for coronary angiography," *Nursing and Midwifery Studies* 3 (2014), e17518.

Erdil, F, and Özhan Elbaş, N, ed. Cerrahi Hastalıkları Hemşireliği. [Surgical Diseases Nursing] 5th ed. (Ankara, Aydoğdu Ofset, 2008), 123-136.

Ledowski, T et al., "Effects of acute postoperative pain on catecholamine plasma levels, hemodynamic parameters, and cardiac autonomic control," *Pain* 153 (2012), 759-764.

Oktay, A.A, et al., "Knowledge Levels of The Vital Signs of Nursing Students," *KSU Medical Journal* 12 (2017), 21-27.

Renn, C.L and Leslie T, *"Relieving Pain and Providing Comfort,"* in Critical Care Nursing Holistic Approach, ed. Morton P.G, Fontaine D.K 10th ed. (Lippincott Williams & Wilkins, 2012), 51-55.

Siedlecki, S.L. "Pain and Sedation", in *AACN Advanced Critical Care Nursing*, 1st ed. ed. Carlson K.K. (Mosby, 2009), 44-52.

Smeltzer, S.C. Bare, B.G, Hinkle J.L, Cheever. K.H. *Brunner & Suddarth's Textbook of Medical-Surgical Nursing.* 12th ed. (Philadelphia, Lippincott Williams & Wilkins, 2010), 756-762.

Younessi, Heravi, M.A., Yaghubi, M., Joharinia, S, "Effect of Change in Patient's Bed Angles on Pain After Coronary Angiography According to Vital Signals," *Journal of Research in Medical Sciences* 20 (2017), 937-943.

White, L, Duncan G, Baumle W. Medical-Surgical Nursing: An Integrated Approach, 3rd ed. Chapter 13, *Caring for Surgical Clients.* (Delmar, Cengage Learning, 2013), 273-300.

In: Vital Signs: An Overview
Editors: Roy Abi Zeid Daou et al.
ISBN: 978-1-53617-765-7
© 2020 Nova Science Publishers, Inc.

Chapter 3

PREDICTION AND DETECTION OF EPILEPSY SEIZURES USING ELECTROPHYSIOLOGICAL MEASUREMENTS

Nashaat El Halabi[1], Roy Abi Zeid Daou[2,3], Roger Achkar[1], Ali Hayek[4] and Josef Boercsoek[4]

[1]American University of Science and Technology, Faculty of Engineering, Department of Computer and Communications Engineering, Beirut, Lebanon
[2]Lebanese German University, Public Health Faculty, Biomedical Technologies Department, Jounieh, Lebanon
[3]Mart, Learning, Education and Research Center, Chananiir, Lebanon
[4]Kassel University, Institute of Computer Architecture and System Programming, Kassel, Germany

ABSTRACT

Epilepsy is a neurological disorder associated with abnormal electrical activity in the brain, which causes seizures. The occurrence of seizures is not predictable; the duration between seizures, as well as the symptoms, varies from patient to patient. Since seizures are not predictable, and most epileptic patients suffer from physical risky symptoms during the seizure, such patients are not able to perform daily work activities.

The objective of this project is to design and implement a monitoring system for epileptic patients; the system should continuously check some vital signs, analyze the measurements, and decide whether the patient is to have a seizure. Whenever a seizure is predicted, the system initiates an alarm. In addition, a notification should be sent to the healthcare responsible, as well as one preferred contact. By implementing the monitoring system, epilepsy patients will have a better chance to work and live a normal life.

The first part of this chapter presents the concept of the overall system and shows the results of the basic system design, which is based on: Electro-Encephalo-Gram (EEG), Electro-Cardio-Gram (ECG) and Fall Detection system. The results have shown that the accuracy of the fall detection system reached 99.89% whereas the accuracy of the prediction using Artificial Neural Networks (ANN) was about 97.34%.

The second part presents the advanced system's architecture: Five classification methods were studied; Decision Trees, Discriminant Analysis, Support Vector Machine (SVM), K-Nearest Neighbor (KNN), and Ensemble Learning. For each of the classification methods, the following measures were studied and compared: the accuracy, the specificity, the sensitivity, the precision, the false detection rate and the F-measure. The results for seizure prediction system have shown that the highest accuracy, specificity and F-Measure, and the lowest false detection rate were achieved with Bagged Trees Ensemble Learning, the highest sensitivity and precision were achieved with Quadratic Support Vector Machine. However, for seizure detection system, the highest accuracy and F-Measure were achieved with Linear Support Vector Machine, the highest sensitivity and specificity were achieved with Fine Gaussian Support Vector Machine, and the highest precision and lowest false detection rate were achieved with Subspace Discriminant Ensemble Learning.

Keywords: neurological disorder, epileptic seizure, electrophysiological signals, accelerometers, Artificial Neural Networks, Decision Trees, Discriminant Analysis, SVM, KNN, Ensemble Learning

INTRODUCTION

Every year, neurodegenerative disorders affect millions of people worldwide. Each disorder presents various health hazards and unpredictable risks, and can often result in the individual having difficulty maintaining a stable life.

While neurodegenerative disorders range in symptoms, they are all characterized by the progressive and irreversible depletion of neurons from specific regions of the brain. The term encompasses a vast range of clinical diseases, including dementia and disordered cognitive function, disabled motor impairment, excessive and abnormal movement, progressive muscle atrophy and epilepsy. This irreversible loss of neurons often, if not always, culminates in death for the patient. Many reasons can lead to the development of the disease, some of them are anxiety and stress due to the disintegration of the patient in workplaces as well as the difficulties in performing their daily life activities. However, it is ultimately the neuronal degeneration itself that causes tragic and unfixable neurological and behavioral disabilities, ranging from complete memory loss to paralysis [1].

Epilepsy is a neurodegenerative disorder that includes symptoms of recurring seizures and psychic symptoms such as anxiety or Deja vu. These seizures, often referred to as fits, are defined as a sudden burst of electrical activity in the brain. Depending on which part of the brain is involved, seizures affect patients in different ways. Seizures vary in gravity, but are by definition characterized by the jerking and shaking of the body. Furthermore, more extreme seizures can include a momentary loss of awareness or unusual sensations, lasting from few seconds to several minutes. Seizures are divided into classes that are identified based on the following criteria: the first one depends on where their inception originates in the brain, which leads to focal or generalized seizures, the second criterion is related to whether or not a person's awareness is affected, and the third depends on whether or not seizures induce sudden movement or loss of movement. Patients diagnosed with epilepsy can face daily problems. Concern and anxiety of an upcoming fit can threaten any stability the individual may hope to have [1].

According to the World Health Organization (WHO), up to June 2019, epilepsy is one of the most common neurodegenerative disorders attacking about 50 million patients worldwide, 80% of them live in low- and middle-income countries. The risk of premature death for people suffering from epilepsy is up to three times higher than healthy people [2].

Treatments for neurodegenerative disorders are considered case-by-case, but the two major forms focus on the restoration of dopaminergic activity or the reduction of cholinergic activity. While researchers have been working hard to find cures in neurodegenerative disorders, there have been little strides to produce conclusive and thoroughly successful results for all cases. By studying early onset signs, researchers are now switching their focus to find solutions and preventive measures to lessen the gravity of a patient's upcoming onset [1].

According to the Epilepsy Foundation, epilepsy patients face many problems in their daily life activities, these problems include feeling uncomfortable at home, work, school and in social activities. They face learning difficulties which makes them in need for special help, they suffer from depression and anxiety, and for sure they feel unsafe while working in industrial environment and while driving [3][2].

In this era of technological evolution, many devices, monitoring systems and phone applications have been developed to help people with various health problems, and have dramatically improved the living conditions for many individuals. However, there is still a lack of solutions for people living with neurodegenerative disorders. For people diagnosed with epilepsy, there remains an absence of complete solution, therefore withholds these individuals from attaining a higher quality of life. As patients can often find it difficult to fully succeed in the work domain, career opportunities, and daily life activities, it is imperative that solutions must be created. While the need for solutions has been discussed, there remains a need for a definitive and all-encompassing solution [3, 2].

During the initial brainstorming, many questions were asked that helped shape and frame the groundwork of the eventual product. How can a system allow people experiencing epilepsy to live a more stable life? If neurodegenerative diseases are not curable, what are tangible ways to enhance the lives of people with epilepsy? What are the high-risk daily activities faced by individuals with epilepsy? How can this product allow users to have a stable work life and flourish in the workforce? As epilepsy itself remains incurable, what other options are there for epileptic patients? And the most challenging key question is how to achieve these objectives in a non-invasive method, without involving the introduction of instruments into the body?

As the questions were formulated and then answered, it became apparent that a device was needed to monitor the patient. The most effective monitoring system would be an easily wearable system that is comfortable for the patient and compatible with all the sensors needed. Moreover, rather than focusing on a treatment to cure epilepsy, it was deemed more practical and safer to create a tool that facilitates the difficulties that the epileptic patients may face.

The Epilepsy Monitoring and detection System Using Wearable Devices is a monitoring system that is worn by the individual and includes sensors that constantly scan to see if there are irregularities in the user's heart and brain activities. If irregularities are detected, the monitoring system will notify the individual and a healthcare professional that a seizure may take place.

The proposed system is a tool for epilepsy patients, engineered to further their ability to excel in society and the workforce. Due to the seizure prediction feature, users of the device can remain assured that a medical assistance will be summoned if a seizure is nearly to take place. The features of the proposed system include, but are not limited to:

prediction and detection of epilepsy seizures: three epilepsy phases are defined, normal phase when no seizure is occurring or about to occur, preictal phase when a seizure is about to occur in few seconds, and ictal phase when a seizure is occurring; detection of a fall using other wearable sensors; sending alerts to specific persons, preselected emergency contact, and a medical professional of the imminent and approaching seizure via a complementary mobile application.

The fundamental goal of the system is to give epileptic patients not only a way to cope with their disease, but also a tool to allow them to thrive in society without feeling socially isolated or ostracized. The system will equip users with a set of wearable sensors that are sewn into the lining of their clothes. The sensors are connected to microcontrollers and then linked to a mobile phone application. By tracking the electrical brain and heart activities, as well as physical gesture, the proposed system will then alert the supervisor and the healthcare provider if an employee may have a seizure approaching. If a fit is underway, an immediate push notification will be sent to the patient's healthcare providers and a preselected emergency contact at the time of occurrence.

Figure 1 shows a block diagram for the whole system. The sensors are the EEG electrodes to read the electrical brain activity, the ECG electrodes to read the electrical heart activity, and the accelerometers to acquire the patient's posture. The EEG and ECG signals are amplified and filtered before being converted from analog to digital form, and features are extracted in parallel with posture analysis from the accelerometers. The main processing unit performs the machine learning algorithm as well as the fall detection algorithm; these two algorithms give three possible outputs for seizure (normal, preictal and ictal), and two possible outputs for fall detection. The notification is initiated in case of ictal, preictal and/or fall detected.

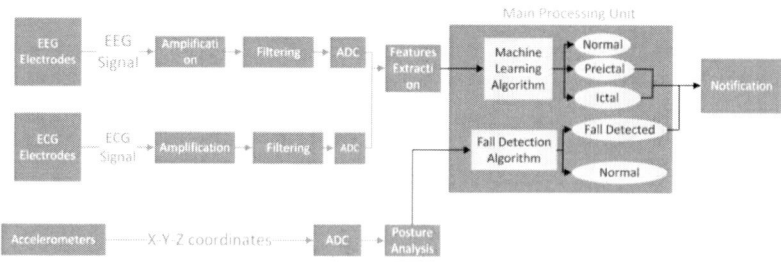

Figure 1. Block Diagram.

Figure 2 shows a simple UML chart for the project as a whole; first, the sensors acquire the analog signals, these signals are then converted from analog to digital. The sampled signals are then processed to extract specific features that will be sent to Classification/Detection/Prediction unit which will then return the actual status of the patient: Normal, Preictal, and Ictal. In case of preictal or ictal states, a push notification will be sent in order to immediately notify the designated healthcare provider via the mobile application.

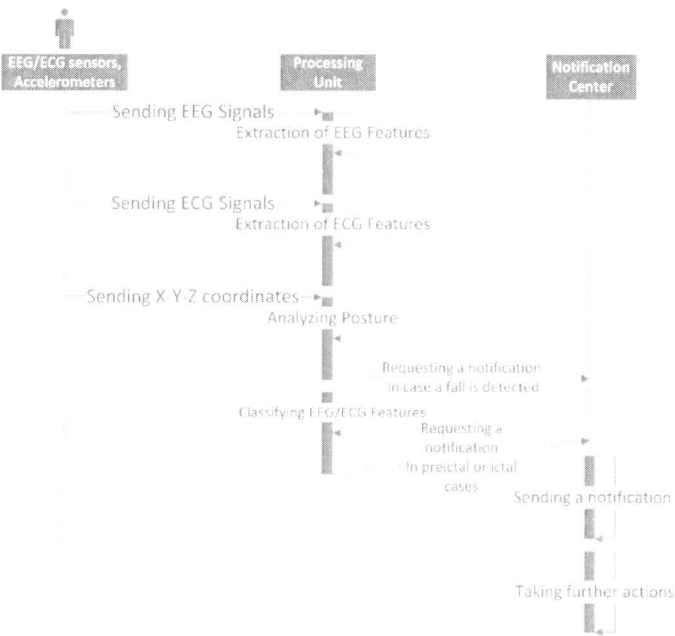

Figure 2. UML chart of the process.

This book chapter will be divided as following: in section 2, the state of the art is discussed and grouped into artificial intelligence simulation methods and vital signs monitoring and analysis. In section 3, the basic system design is discussed, where the whole system is described and the testing of electrophysiology subsystem as well as the fall detection subsystem is discussed. Section 4 shows the advanced system processing, including the five classification methods and their results. And finally section 5 includes the conclusions and future work.

2. STATE OF THE ART

Different types of systems and applications have been introduced to help epilepsy patients. Their uses range from imparting general information about epilepsy, teaching first aid and safety methods when a sudden seizure occurs, and/or providing self-monitoring tools. This section describes the literature review including systems and research studies that are related to epilepsy, it includes studies related to seizure detection, seizure prediction and fall detection.

In 2015, a SmartWatch was developed by Patterson and his research group to alert patients when unusual movements were detected [4]. In 2014, another device, developed by Eftekhar et al., was designed to look like a cap; it is to be worn by patients at all times in order to monitor their brainwaves [5]. In 2015, a team at Vanderbilt University Medical Center has created another method to treat epilepsy through surgery. This method employs an MRI-guided laser ablation in order to destroy the brain tissues causing seizures in place of surgical resection [6]. In 2017, a mother developed a product for her epileptic son in India; she designed a glove with sensors sewn where various vitals from the body could be measured [7].

For a long time, the diagnosis of epilepsy, as well as detection and prediction of its seizures, has been an important and challenging domain for researchers. Many scientists have been working on using biosensors to detect seizures; however, prediction has been always a more complicated and difficult task because seizures are recurrent and unpredictable.

2.1. Detection of Epilepsy Seizure

This part presents some of the previous projects that aimed to detect epilepsy seizures. In 2010, Sorensen et al. have proposed a system for onset detection of epilepsy seizures using EEG features. The dataset consisted of EEG recordings from six patients; it included 133 seizures in a total recording time of 305 hours. Two of the patients had sEEG (scalp EEG) recordings, and the other four patients had iEEG (intracranial EEG) recordings. All EEG recordings were sampled at a sampling frequency of 200 Hz[8] [8]. The proposed system combined the Matching Pursuit algorithm and the Support Vector Machine (SVM) as feature extractor and classifier, respectively; two features were extracted from the EEG signals, the *Gabor Atom Density* (GAD) and the *Mean Atom Frequency* (MAF). The proposed system achieved a sensitivity of 78–100%, a False Detection Rate (FDR) of 0.16–5.31 per hour and a detection latency of 5–18s. The detailed results are shown in Table 1 [8].

Table 1. Sorensen et al. Results Summary [8]

Patient	NB. Of Seizures	Sensitivity (%)	FDR (1/h)	Latency (s)
P1	10	100	0.59	18.3
P2	49	91.4	5.31	9.1
P3	35	NA	NA	NA
P4	20	95	0.20	6.06
P5	13	77.8	0.16	5.67
P6	6	100	1.8	7.44

In 2011, Kharbouch et al. used a patient-specific algorithm for epileptic seizure onset binary detection; the algorithm classified intracranial EEG recordings into ictal and non-ictal. The algorithm extracted features from intracranial spectral and temporal electroencephalography. The features consisted of the spectral distribution of iEEG, the channels on which it manifests, and its short-term temporal evolution. In order to extract the spectral features, the researchers applied multiple filters to a sliding window and they found the energy within the passband of each filter. Then, automated machine learning based on Linear Support Vector Machine (LSVM) was performed to detect unrecognized events as well as seizures. Out of 67 seizure tests, the algorithm detected 97% with a detection delay of 5s and a false alarm rate of 0.6 per 24-hour period. The authors state that their proposed system solved the problem of heterogeneity of seizure iEEG readings between patients and sometimes with the same patient [9].

Also in 2011, Acharya et al. have used nonlinear Higher Order Spectra (HOS) features in order to classify ECG readings as normal, preictal and ictal. The ECG signal was used first to detect the peaks QRS and the time interval between them, and then Cumulant Computation was applied in addition to Discrete Wavelet Transform (DWT) followed by Principal component analysis (PCA) statistical analysis in order to get the features that would be fed to the Artificial Neural Networks (ANN) and Support Vector Machine (SVM) for classification. A set of 300 recordings from the three epileptic classes (normal, preictal and ictal) was used. The results showed a detection accuracy of 98.5% with a high confidence level (p-value < 0.0001) [10].

In 2012, Liu et al. proposed a system that automatically detects seizures using wavelet decomposition; the authors used multi-channel intracranial EEG to extract features using Wavelet transform, where iEEG signals were decomposed into three bands, and then the extracted features were the relative energy, the relative amplitude, the coefficient of variation and the fluctuation index. The features were then sent to SVM for classification. Post-processing steps were performed as well; these steps included smoothing, multi-channel decision fusion and collar technique. The proposed system achieved a sensitivity of 94.46%, a specificity of 95.26%, and a false detection rate of 0.58 per hour [11].

Recently, in 2017, Wang et al. presented a system for epilepsy seizure detection based on combining Discrete Wavelet Transform (DWT) and the nonlinear Sparse Extreme Learning Machine (SELM). The proposed system was a three-classes classifier. The authors decomposed the EEG signals into four known bands: delta (ranging from 0 to 4 Hz), theta (ranging from 4 to 8 Hz), alpha (ranging from 8 to 16 Hz) and beta (ranging from 16 to 32 Hz). This decomposition was applied by three-levels lifting DWT using Daubechies order-4 wavelet. The algorithm started by training the dataset, where features were extracted using Lifting based Discrete Wavelet Transform (LDWT). And then, the features were sent for learning using SELM, thus creating the EEG Classification Models (Multiclass SELM) that were used for testing later on. The authors stated that their system achieved high classification accuracy and short training and testing time, where after using CHB-MIT dataset (will be defined later on in this section), the sensitivity of the binary SELM was 81.1% and the specificity was 98.3% [12].

In 2011, Petersen et al. studied the detection of epilepsy seizures using single channel sEEG. The system was studied with a dataset consisting of 24 recordings from 19 patients, with a total duration of 11 hours and 48 minutes, containing a total of 177 seizures. The recordings were sampled at 200 Hz, and band-pass filters with a passband of 0.53-70 Hz were applied. For features extraction, the researchers have used wavelet transform in order to get the energy of the different sub-bands. The classification has been done using SVM adjusted lately by temporal constraints. The best results were obtained with the channel F7-FP1, where the sensitivity was 99.1% and the false detection rate was 0.5/h [13].

In 2013, Borujeny et al. investigated in epilepsy seizure detection based on the physical movement of the patient. Thus, a wearable sensor network was created based on 2D accelerometer sensors that monitor the patient posture continuously, and the extracted features are the variance and the correlation of the accelerometers' readings. Three accelerometers were placed on the right arm, left arm and left thigh respectively. The dataset includes 20 epileptic seizures, recorded from 3 patients at a sampling frequency of 3 Hz, and a sliding window of 9 seconds. The authors studied the use of Artificial Neural Networks (ANN) and k-Nearest Neighbor (KNN) algorithms in order to differentiate between seizure or non-seizure movements. The results have shown that KNN achieved better results in terms of false alarm. By using ANN, 15% of the marked seizures were not detected. However, by using KNN, 100% of the marked seizures were detected [14].

In 2019, Wang et al. combined multi-domain features extraction and nonlinear analysis of EEG signals in order to detect epileptic seizures. The features are extracted from time domain, frequency domain, time-frequency domain and non-linear analysis based on information theory. The features are extracted after preprocessing of EEG signals and applying Principal component analysis (PCA); thus, the features included the standard deviation, the total variation, the relative power from Fast Fourier

Transform (FFT), the standard deviation and relative power from DWT, the entropy, and the Min-Max-Mean from DWT coefficients. Wavelet Threshold Denoising technique with the fourth-order Daubechies (db4) was used in order to decompose the EEG signal into its main five sub-bands. The wavelet features were extracted later in order to be inputs for the classifiers. The authors combined multiple classifiers to detect Epileptic seizures: K-Nearest Neighbor (KNN), Linear Discriminant Analysis (LDA), Naive Bayesian (NB), Logistic Regression (LR) and Support Vector Machine (SVM). The proposed system achieved an average accuracy of 99.25% [15].

2.2. Prediction of Epilepsy Seizure

The following part presents some of the previous projects that predicted epilepsy seizures:

In 2010, Chisci et al. have implemented a system for epileptic seizure detection and prediction; although the title of their research is "Real-Time Epileptic Seizure Prediction Using AR Models and Support Vector Machines", the authors investigated the binary classification of epileptic seizures, which means that they combined ictal and pre-ictal classes into one class, and normal (or inter-ictal) class is the second class. The system is based on estimating the least-squares parameter from the time domain representation of EEG, and using SVM for classification. The authors used the Freiburg dataset and applied the Kalman filter within the SVM process. As the authors stated, their system achieved 100% sensitivity and low false detection rate [16].

In 2014, Teixeira et al. developed and implemented a hardware named Brainatic for real-time scalp EEG-based epileptic seizure prediction. The system applies machine learning methods for real-time prediction of seizures; it extracts 22 features from each EEG electrode, and classifies the readings using support vector machines, Multi-Layer Perceptron (MLP) neural networks and Radial Basis Functions (RBF) neural networks. The system, named Brainatic, has been implemented with a dual Intel®

Atom™ netbook with 2GB of RAM to facilitate the process of computing the features from EEG real-time recordings. This hardware has been used to perform the clinical tests for the European project EPILEPSIAE [17].

Table 2. Researches on Prediction of Epilepsy Seizures

Authors	Year of Research	Dataset	Features	Classifier	Sensitivity
Maiwald et al. [19]	2004	FB^1	Dynamical similarity index	Threshold crossing	42
Winterhalder et al. [20]	2006	FB^1	Phase coherence lag synchronization	Threshold crossing	60
Park et al. [21]	2011	FB^1	Univariate spectral power	SVM	98.3
Gadhoumi et al. [22]	2012	MNI^2	Wavelet energy, entropy	Discriminant Analysis	88.9
Li et al. [23]	2013	FB^1	Spike rate	Threshold crossing	72.7
Zheng et al. [24]	2014	FB^1	Mean phase coherence	Threshold crossing	>70
Eftekhar et al. [5]	2014	FB^1	Multiresolution N-gram	Threshold crossing	90.95
Aarabi et al. [25]	2014	FB^1	Bayesien inversion of power spectral density	Rule-based decision	87.07
Zhang et al. [26]	2016	FB^1	Power spectral density ratio	SVM	100
Parvez et al. [27]	2017	FB^1	Phase-match error, deviation, fluctuation	SVM	95.4
Sharif et al. [28]	2017	FB^1	Fuzzy rules on Poincare plane	SVM	91.8-96.6
Aarabi et al. [29]	2017	FB^1	Univariate and bivariate features	Rule-based decision	86.7

1: Freiburg Hospital intracranial EEG (iEEG) dataset.
2: Montreal Neurological Institute intracranial EEG (iEEG) dataset.

In 2014, Parvez and Paul have developed a system for epileptic seizure prediction by extracting several features from the different EEG bands and applying the DWT (Daubechies order 4-wavelet - db4) in order to decompose the EEG signal into its five main bands. The authors used a dataset from the University Hospital of Freiburg, Germany. It consists of recordings from 21 patients, sampled at 256 Hz with a 16-bits analog to digital converter. SVM was used for classification; two classes were defined, pre-ictal and inter-ictal. The authors state that applying their method and decomposing EEG readings into its different bands made their system more sensitive, specific and accurate compared to the previously implemented systems for classification of EEG readings and prediction of seizures, thus their results have shown an accuracy of 95.34% [18].

Many other researchers have been working on the prediction of epileptic seizures using intracranial EEG (iEEG). Table 2 shows the contributions along with the different parameters considered in the studies and the obtained sensitivity.

2.3. Researches on CHB-MIT Dataset

Many researchers have been working on using EEG/ECG datasets for detection and prediction of Epileptic seizures; however, few of them studied "user-specified" classification, such that the system will be trained specifically for a unique patient, and the dataset for learning is individually studied. For this purpose, a database from Massachusetts Institute of Technology (referred lately as CHB-MIT) [30] has been used for ECG and EEG signals, and time/frequency domain features have been extracted and used for classification. The database consists of 5 seconds segments sampled at a sampling frequency of 256 Hz.

Since CHB-MIT dataset will be used for the simulation and the validation of the proposed system mentioned in this chapter, the following is a short description of some works done by researchers who have chosen the same dataset for classification of epileptic EEG/ECG recordings. Some of the projects study "cross patient seizure" which means the detection and/or prediction is not patient-specific, and others study "patient-specific" detection and/or prediction.

In 2009, Shoeb used SVM with spectral, spatial and temporal features in order to design patient-specific seizure detection and prediction system. His study has achieved a sensitivity of 96% after using CHB-MIT dataset [31]. With the same dataset, in 2016, Zabihi et al. have used Linear Discriminant Analysis (LDA) and Naive Bayesian classification for the same purpose, which is patient-specific seizure detection. Their project achieved a sensitivity of 88.27% and a specificity of 93.21% [32].

In 2014, Hills was able to achieve an accuracy of 96% for epilepsy patient-specific seizure detection after using Random Forests classification that has been processed on Fast Fourier Transform of EEG/ECG recordings [33]. In 2016, Fergus et al. applied KNN classification method for statistical features extracted from the same dataset in order to solve the problem of cross patient epilepsy seizure detection. The applied method has shown an accuracy of 93% and a sensitivity of 88% [34].

In 2015, Xun et al. used Sparse Autoencoders and SVM for classification of temporal features extracted from CHB-MIT dataset for the purpose of patient-specific epileptic seizure classification; their study has achieved an accuracy of 88.8% [35]. Similarly, in 2017, Chen et al. have presented a seizure detection algorithm based on Discrete Wavelet Transform (DWT) and EEG from CHB-MIT dataset and UBonn dataset. Their design and their classification method have achieved an accuracy of 92.30% with the first dataset, and 99.33% with the second [36].

In 2014, Siddharth et al. used feed-forward Neural Networks by applying leave-one-out cross-validation on the CHB–MIT dataset. The study achieved a sensitivity of 98% and an accuracy of 78% for cross patient epilepsy seizure classification [37][37]. Also, in the same year, Turner et al. achieved an accuracy of 90% for cross patient epilepsy seizure classification after using KNN, SVM and logistic regression classifications. The researchers deployed deep belief networks in multichannel and high-resolution EEG data with CHB-MIT dataset [38].

In 2017, Ye et al. investigated using Short-Time Fourier Transform (STFT) with stacked denoising auto encoders to study patient-specific seizure classification. They were able to achieve an accuracy of 98% on the CHB–MIT dataset [39]. Similarly, in 2014, Akara et al. used logistic classifiers with stacked auto encoders and tested their method on CHB–MIT dataset. The researchers declared that their method has shown a latency of 3.36 seconds and a low false detection rate (below 0.00 per hour) [40]. Also, in 2016, for the purpose of cross-patient epileptic seizure detection, Thodoroff et al. used recurrent convolution deep Neural Networks to extract features of seizures from the CHB–MIT dataset. Their method achieved a sensitivity of 85% [41]. More recently, in 2018, Ghulam et al. used Convolutional Neural Networks and applied it on CHB-MIT dataset for a cross-patient epilepsy classification algorithm. The researchers have achieved an accuracy of 99.02% and a sensitivity of 92.35% [42].

2.4. Researches on Fall Detection

Creating fall detection systems has been a widely studied topic throughout the past years. Such systems can be camera based systems, ambient sensors based systems, and wearable sensors based systems. The common fall detection systems are based on the following step-by-step procedure: first, data is collected using specific sensors, then the features are selected and extracted from the data in order to be sent to the classifier, and finally the results are analyzed in order to detect falls [43].

Starting by the sensors, they can be wearable [44] [44-60], which make them able to be embedded in other monitoring devices. The commonly used sensors are the accelerometers, the gyroscopes, wearable cameras and some health sensors like the Electromyogram (EMG) sensors. The sensors can also be ambient sensors [61-3], and they can be camera-based sensors [74-88].

In addition, the fall detection systems use different algorithms for classification, threshold based algorithms and Machine Learning algorithms are commonly used. Table 3 shows some projects and studies related to fall detection and monitoring.

Table 3. Researches on Fall Detection

Reference	Sensors Type	Sensors	Classifier	Accuracy (%)	Sensitivity (%)	Specificity (%)	Precision (%)
[44]	Wearable sensors	Smartphone compass, accelerometer, proximity, gyroscope	Decision tree, SVM	90			
[45]	Wearable sensors	Accelerometer	Comparator System	99			
[46]	Wearable sensors	Accelerometer, pressure sensor, Smartphone	State Machine				
[47]	Wearable sensors	Accelerometer	Health level fuzzy petri net	90			
[48]	Wearable sensors	Electromyography	Decision Tree		83.2	72.4	
[49]	Wearable sensors	Accelerometer	Gaussian mixture model	91.15			
[50]	Wearable sensors	Smartphone camera	Decision Tree	93.78			
[51]	Wearable sensors	Accelerometer, gyroscope, barometric altimeter	Decision Tree		80	100	
[52]	Wearable sensors	Accelerometer, gyroscope	KNN		95	96.67	
[53]	Wearable sensors	Smartphone compass accelerometer	SVM, State Machine		92	99.75	
[54]	Wearable sensors	Accelerometer, cardio tachometer	Decision Tree	97.5	96.8	98.1	
[55]	Wearable sensors	Accelerometer	Binary structure classifier	95.6			
[56]	Wearable sensors	Accelerometer	One Class SVM	96.7			
[57]	Wearable sensors	Gyroscope	Decision Tree			100	
[58]	Wearable sensors	Accelerometer	Decision Tree		98		
[59]	Wearable sensors	Accelerometer	Decision Tree	92.92			
[60]	Wearable sensors	Accelerometer, barometric pressure	Decision Tree	96.9	97.5	96.5	
[61]	Ambient Sensors	PIR and vibration	SVM	100			
[62]	Ambient Sensors	Vibration and microphone	Naive Bayes		97.5	98.6	

Table 3. (Continued)

Reference	Sensors Type	Sensors	Classifier	Accuracy (%)	Sensitivity (%)	Specificity (%)	Precision (%)
[63]	Ambient Sensors	Circular microphone array	KNN		100	97	
[64]	Ambient Sensors	Doppler and motion sensors	SVM				
[65]	Ambient Sensors	Accelerometer and microphone	Gaussian mixture model		95	95	
[66]	Ambient Sensors	Microphone	One class support vector machine	90.63			
[67]	Ambient Sensors	Special Piezo transducer	Pattern matching		95	95	
[68]	Ambient Sensors	Far-Field microphone	SVM				70
[69]	Ambient Sensors	Accelerometer	Decision Tree		87	97.7	
[70]	Ambient Sensors	Piezo resistive pressure sensor	Decision Tree		88.8	94.9	
[71]	Ambient Sensors	PIR	Hidden Markov model	80			
[72]	Ambient Sensors	Doppler	KNN	93.3			
[73]	Ambient Sensors	Electric near-field	Two-state Markov chain		91		
[74]	Camera-Based	Depth sensor	Decision Tree	93	94	91.3	
[75]	Camera-Based	RGB	SVM	93.38			
[76]	Camera-Based	Kinect and accelerometer	Fuzzy interference and decision tree	98.38			
[77]	Camera-Based	Kinect	Decision Tree				94.31
[78]	Camera-Based	Kinect and accelerometer	SVM	98.33	100		94.6
[79]	Camera-Based	Wide angle camera	SVM	97			
[80]	Camera-Based	Kinect	Decision Tree	98.7			
[81]	Camera-Based	RGB	Decision Tree		99.7	99.7	
[82]	Camera-Based	RGB	Decision Tree		88	87.5	
[83]	Camera-Based	RGB	One class support vector machine	100			
[84]	Camera-Based	3D	Decision Tree	78.9			
[85]	Camera-Based	RGB	Gaussian multi-frame	85			
[86]	Camera-Based	RGB	Multi-class support vector machine		90.27	95.16	
[87]	Camera-Based	RGB	String matching	96			
[88]	Camera-Based	RGB	Decision tree	90			

3. BASIC SYSTEM DESIGN

This project aims to develop a monitoring and decision-making system for epilepsy patients, in order to offer them a stable life in which they will be able to work and pursue daily activities with ease, not fearing an upcoming onset. By giving them peace of mind, we hope to also quell the concerns of their families.

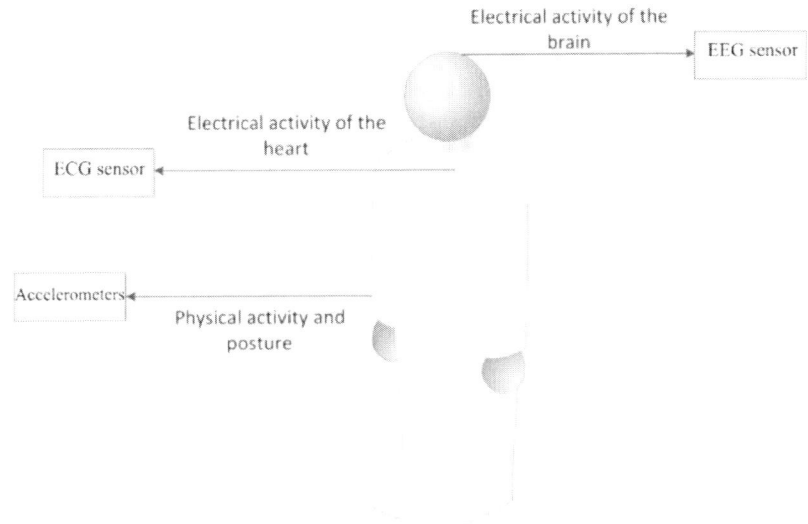

Figure 3. Sensors used for the proposed system.

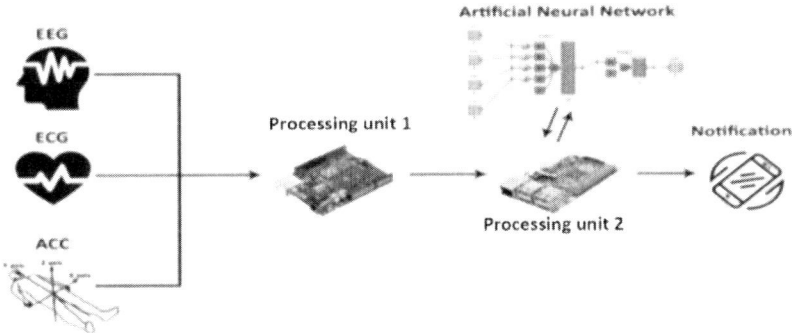

Figure 4. Block diagram of the complete system.

As for the applied tools, the monitoring of the epilepsy patients will be done by recording their vital signs using three types of sensors: the ECG (Electrocardiogram), the EEG (Electroencephalogram) and the accelerometers. The first sensor will record the cardiac activity whereas the second one is used to identify the brain's activity. Both sensors will be applied for the prediction of the seizure using advanced processing tools like the ones listed in the previous section, mainly the neural networks, the machine learning and the signal processing tools. As for the accelerometers, they will be used to detect the fall of the patient as well as his/her current activity. Figure 3 shows the placements of these sensors (concerning the accelerometer, three sensors were implemented as will be shown later on) whereas Figure 4 shows the interconnection of the three sensors using some processing units.

Several measures were considered when choosing the sensors: the cost of the system, its accuracy, its comfort and its ease of use were the major issues. For that, we were limited to the use of three types of sensors only. A seizure is predicted if at least 1 of the 2 used electrophysiological systems delivers a notification. As for the detection, at least 2 out of the 3 sensors must identify the seizure in order to initiate an alarm.

In case of a seizure, the system must detect the exact location of the patient using a GPS sensor. And then, It sends a notification to the parents of the patient, as well as his/her healthcare provider, via a phone application.

Figure 5 shows the flowchart of the whole system. The signals, coming from the sensors, are inputted to the first processing unit, in this case the Arduino, to be converted from analog to digital form. The resulting outputs will be transferred to another microcontroller, the raspberry Pi, using the I^2C communication protocol, for signal manipulation as the latter enables the communication with the ANN. The ANN is applied using Matlab® and delivers one of the three following outputs: Normal, Preictal, and Ictal. In case a preictal or an ictal state is detected, a notification will be sent to the designated healthcare provider via the mobile phone application.

As for the implementation, three Arduino microcontrollers are used, each connected to one or more sensors. Although this big number would lead to additional data transmission risks, the main focus in this design is to have a functional system. As for the Raspberry pi, only one device will be deployed. It will serve as the central processing unit for the whole system.

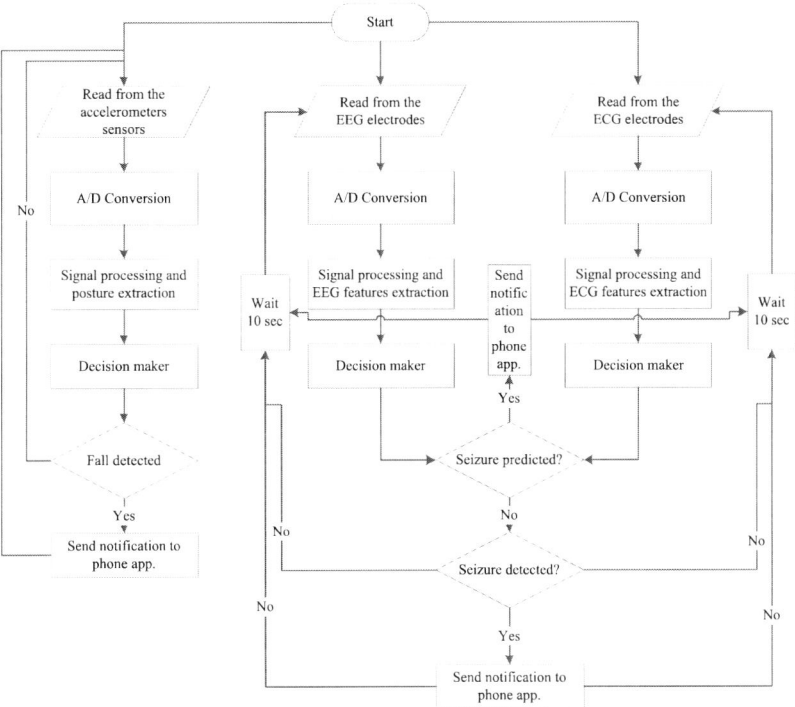

Figure 5. Flowchart for complete system.

Going into more details concerning Figure 3, the clothing design used is an overall that could be easily wearable by anyone. After proper calibration, the three accelerometers will be continuously reading in order to detect a fall. Two EEG electrodes are embedded in a headband along with one electrode beneath the ear for grounding. As for the ECG, three electrodes are used: two connected to the chest and the third connected to the leg. The readings are transmitted through wires that are embedded into the clothing, to the Arduino that is connected to EEG and ECG processing boards, these boards are placed in a sealed pocket on the overall, also the raspberry pi is placed in the same pocket to receive the sampled readings from the Arduino. The last part consists of using a wireless communication module that will notify the phone application user of any occurring or predicted seizure.

Since it is very difficult to test the whole system on real epilepsy patients, the testing phase was divided into two phases; the electrophysiology subsystem was tested using pre-recorded dataset for EEG and ECG signals, and the fall detection subsystem was tested on 5 non-epileptic persons.

3.1. Testing the Electrophysiology Subsystem

In this section, the ECG and the EEG will be presented. The placement of the electrodes for each sensor along with the electronic circuit used to capture, analyze and take the required action will be shown. Before proceeding with each system alone, some common parts were implemented for both sensors as the processing tool, mainly the Artificial Neural Network as well as the signal acquisition and pre-processing from the electrodes, converting the output from an analog form to a digital form and sending it to the second processing unit, the Raspberry pi, for further processing using Matlab® software. Thus, this common part will be presented once before showing the characteristics of each sub-system alone.

To start, the Neural Network Toolbox™ provides algorithms, pre-trained models, and apps to create, train, visualize, and simulate Neural Networks. It offers a classification, regression, clustering, dimensionality reduction, time-series forecasting, and dynamic system modeling and control [89].

This computational tool is one of many that can be used to predict and detect seizures. The first trial was implementing ANN in the Raspberry Pi without having to go through Matlab, but this was not efficient since this algorithm was so heavy on the operating system. By this, testing could not accomplish an acceptable accuracy, and only 77% of testing samples were correctly predicted. Thus, it was a must to implement the ANN on an external server, and send the features to it periodically from Raspberry pi. MATLAB was chosen for its compatibility with Raspberry pi and the Neural Networks Toolbox™ has been used to design and create the ANN, MLP Back propagation algorithm was applied; it adapts the network with weight and bias learning rules according to Levenberg-Marquardt optimization [89].

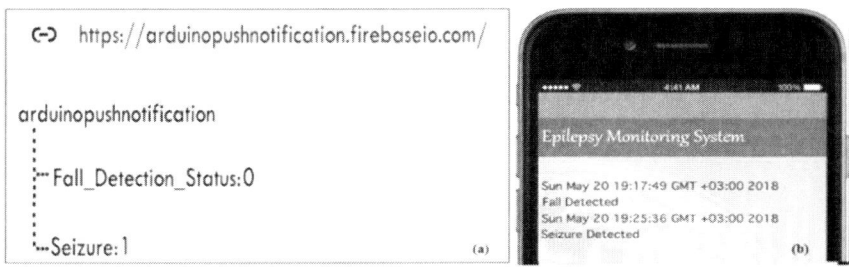

Figure 6. Firebase (a) and mobile (b) interfaces when a seizure a recorder using the electrophysiology devices.

Since testing the system on real epileptic patients is a very difficult task due to the unpredictability of seizures and the non-availability of patients not taking medication, a virtual environment was created; the testing dataset was exported to a Microsoft Excel sheet, and by using PLX-DAQ application, the Arduino randomly chooses one of the samples (since each sample in the dataset is a 10 seconds recording sampled at 256 Hz) and transmits it to the Raspberry pi. Once the recordings are transformed to digital signals using the Arduino (ADC module), with a sampling frequency of 256 Hz (which is compatible with the sampling frequency of the dataset), I^2C connection is initiated between the two Arduino boards (EEG and ECG) and the Raspberry Pi. The sampled recordings are processed at the Raspberry pi level in order to extract the features needed for the ANN. After extracting the features of both signals, the Raspberry Pi uses UDP communication protocol to transmit them to the server running the ANN using a Wi-Fi connection. Based on the processing of the ANN, which gives one out of three outputs: normal, ictal or preictal, the server transmits the decision to the Firebase: a '0' corresponds to normal state, where no notification is needed, and a '1' corresponds to ictal or preictal state, where a notification is generated. In addition, a log is updated in the mobile phone application indicating the time of occurrence and the state; in this case, the message "Seizure detected" is printed out on the screen of the mobile device. Figure 6 shows the Firebase interface and the mobile phone application interface when a seizure is detected.

In the following, the specific parts of each electrophysiological system will be presented.

The procedure for the filtering and amplification of the basic signal coming from the electrodes is shown in Figure 7. The first stage consists of the pre-amplification of the signal. Then, the filtering is needed to keep the useful signal and remove noise and artifacts coming from the movement of the patient and the interference with the power line. A band pass active filter of order 2 is used at this level. The third step consists of a second amplification stage. At this stage, the signal is ready to be sent to the Arduino for an Analog-to-Digital conversion. The last step consists of sending the digitized data to the Raspberry Pi microcontroller that will extract the features of the upcoming signals and sends them to the server station in order to be processed using the ANN.

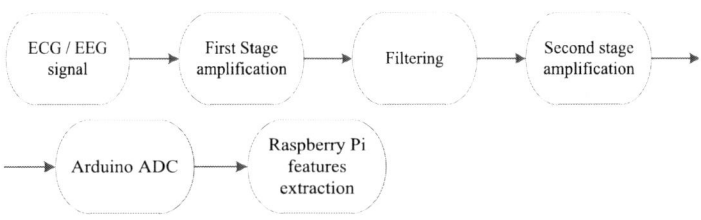

Figure 7. Pre-processing and processing procedure applied for the EEG and ECG signals.

For the EEG signal, the pre-amplification gain is of order 10; the active band pass filter operates between 1 Hz and 130 Hz with a gain of order 220. Two additional gain phases are used as each one of them delivers a gain of 15. The overall gain of the circuit is about 500.000 in order to be able to amplify the input signal from the electrodes from 0-10μV to 0-5V.

After the preprocessing and the analog-to-digital conversion steps, the features extraction is realized on Raspberry pi. As already listed, both the time domain and the frequency domain features will be treated. For the time domain, using a 10 seconds window and 256 Hz sampling rate, the features are the *mean*, the *standard deviation*, and the peak values (*minimum* and *maximum* values). As for the frequency domain features, the EEG signal will be decomposed using Discrete wavelet transform (DWT), into its 5 bands: Delta waves (0.5 to 4 Hz), Theta waves (4 to 8 Hz), Alpha waves (8 to 12 Hz), Beta waves (12 to 30 Hz) and Gamma waves (30+ Hz). These features will be sent later on to the ANN for further processing in order to classify the actual status of the patient.

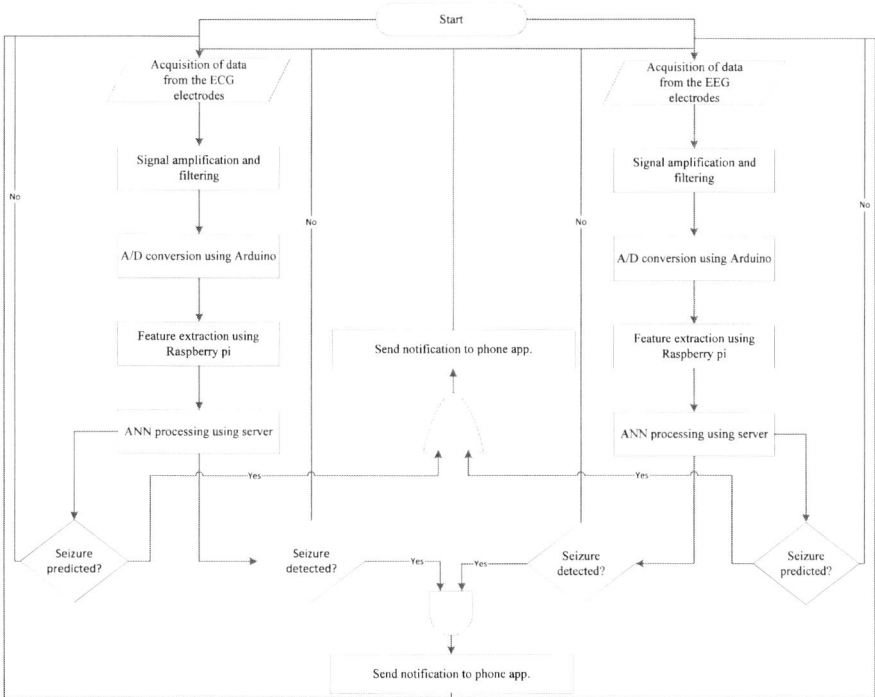

Figure 8. Flowchart of the algorithm used to predict and detect seizures based on the electrophysiological data.

Concerning the ECG system, the same procedure of the EEG is applied. However, the gain factors may vary as the signal is of millivolts order. So, the gain of the first amplification stage is 2.2 whereas the active band pass range applied for the filtering stage is between 1 Hz and 130 Hz.

The post amplification phase for this circuit is not needed; as the overall needed gain is 500, which is assured by the use of the first two stages only.

After being digitized, the signal is transmitted to the Raspberry pi. For this subsystem, only time domain features are computed. The extracted characteristics of the ECG signal are the average heart rate per minute and the mean R-R interval distance.

Not to forget that a notch filter was added for both systems in order to remove the interference of the power line if the patient decides, for some reasons, to connect the devices to the power line and not use a battery.

To conclude this part, Figure 8 represents the flowchart of the electrophysiological algorithm.

3.2. Testing the Fall Detection Subsystem

Several sensors could be used to detect the fall of a pedestrian. However, for this system, the ADXL345 3-axis digital accelerometer is deployed; it is small and thin, which makes it appropriate for wearable systems. It is connected to NODEMCU (ESP8266) in order to initiate a connection between Arduino and Google Firebase to which the Raspberry pi was connected as well.

When a fall is detected, the Firebase launches a notification to the mobile phone application, updates the log in the mobile phone application indicating the time of occurrence and the state that occurred; in this case, it is "Fall detected" message which appears on the phone application.

As for the implementation process, three sensors have been used along with two microcontrollers for processing: the first Arduino is connected to two accelerometers placed next the patient's waist and shoulder, and the second Arduino is connected only to the accelerometer which is placed next to the patient's leg. The use of two microcontrollers can be explained by the fact that one of the objectives of this design is to limit the cost of the system. Thus, as the first two listed accelerometer sensors are near one to the other, only one Arduino was used.

Prediction and Detection of Epilepsy Seizures ...   53

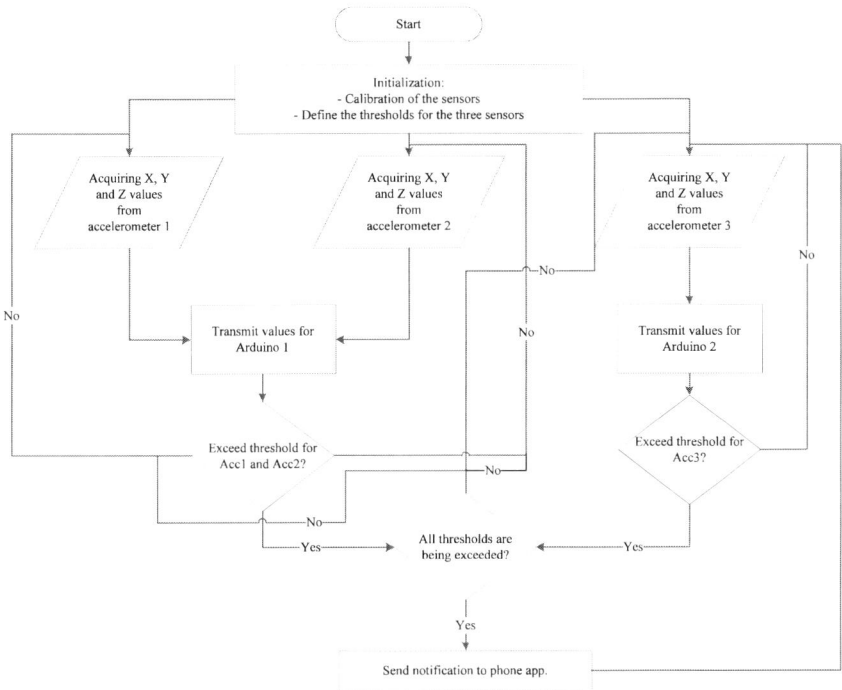

Figure 9. Flowchart of the algorithm used to detect falls applied to the accelerometer system.

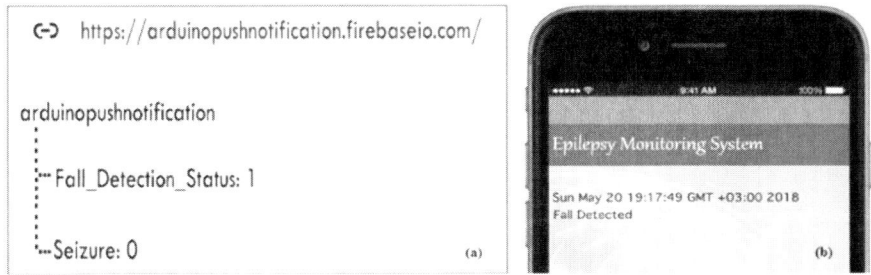

Figure 10. Firebase (a) and mobile (b) interfaces when recoding a fall via the fall detection system.

Concerning the procedure of the fall detection subsystem, a calibration is always needed when initiating at first the system. It consists on defining the threshold values for the sensors that will be considered to identify if a fall has occurred or not. Then, the measurement recording and analysis is performed. After getting the values of the three coordinates X, Y and Z, the sensors send them to the Arduino microcontrollers. If the three sensors find values above the predefined thresholds, a notification is sent to the mobile phone application through the Google firebase. Figure 9 shows the flowchart of the software running to detect falls, whereas figure 10 shows the Firebase interface and the mobile phone application's interface when a fall is detected.

3.3. Results of the Basic System Design

Table 4. CHB-MIT Dataset used for EEG/ECG subsystems

Subject	Gender	Age	Number of seizures	Number of normal samples	Number of preictal samples	Number of ictal samples
1	F	11	7	43	43	43
2	M	11	3	16	16	16
3	F	14	6	38	38	38
4	M	22	4	37	37	37
5	F	7	5	55	55	55
6	F	1.5	10	14	14	14
7	F	14.5	3	32	32	32
8	M	3.5	5	91	91	91
9	F	10	4	33	33	33
10	M	3	7	43	43	43
11	F	12	3	80	80	80
12	F	2	27	95	95	95
13	F	3	2	11	11	11
14	F	9	8	15	15	15
15	M	16	20	196	196	196
16	F	7	8	4	4	4
17	F	12	3	29	29	29
18	F	18	6	31	31	31
19	F	19	3	23	23	23
20	F	6	8	27	27	27
21	F	13	4	14	14	14
22	F	9	3	19	19	19
23	F	6	7	41	41	41
24	NA	NA	16	48	48	48

As the system was still in the realization phase, its application on epileptic patients was not possible. However, each subsystem has been tested alone. A database from Massachusetts Institute of Technology was used [30][30]. The database was reshaped and it consisted of 5 seconds segments sampled at 256 Hz sampling frequency. Table 4 shows some details about the subjects of the dataset. The values and the signals found in the database will be used for testing the algorithms and the overall system. As for the fall detection system, it was fully implemented and tested.

The system has been tested with different features sets. The first step was using time domain features for EEG and ECG signals, which include: mean, standard deviation, maximum and minimum form EEG signals, average heart rate and R-R interval from ECG signals, which result in 1x6 input and 1x1 output for the ANN as shown in Figure 11.

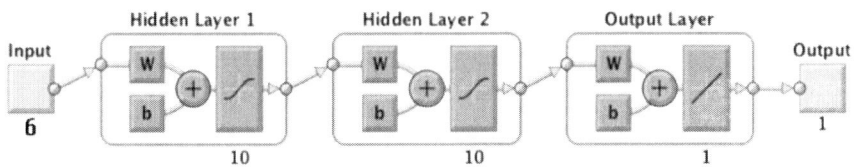

Figure 11. ANN architecture – time domain features.

When training using "Traingdx" method, which updates weight and bias values according to gradient descent momentum and an adaptive learning rate, 2 hidden layers with 10 neurons each achieved training mse (mean square error) of 0.0225. However, when training using "Trainlm" method, which updates weight and bias values according to Levenberg-Marquardt optimization, 2 hidden layers with 10 neurons each achieved best training mse of 0.0196 at epoch 100. When testing the last ANN with time domain features only, the test mse was 0.029, 97.1% of test samples were correctly predicted, 2.9% were incorrectly predicted.

The second step was training the ANN using frequency domain features of EEG signal as shown in Figure 12.

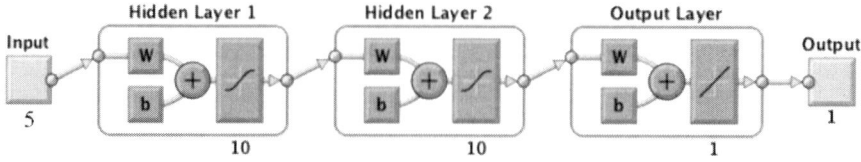

Figure 12. ANN architecture – frequency domain features.

With frequency domain features, using Levenberg-Marquardt optimization, 2 hidden layers with 10 neurons each achieved best training mse of 0.39374 at epoch 100. When testing the last ANN with time domain features only, the test mse was 0.3783, 62.17% of test samples were correctly predicted, 37.83% were incorrectly predicted.

The last step was combining time domain and frequency domain features, so the total number of features is 11, and the ANN architecture is shown in Figure 13.

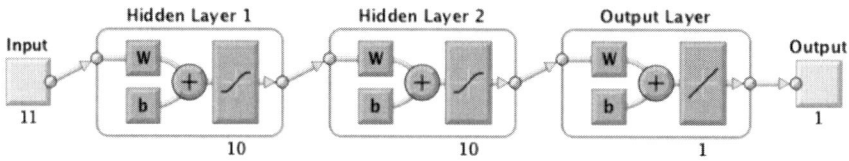

Figure 13. ANN architecture – time/frequency domain features.

With time and frequency domain features, using Levenberg-Marquardt optimization, 2 hidden layers with 10 neurons each achieved best training mse of 0.017177 at epoch 100. When testing the last ANN with time domain features only, the test mse was 0.027667, 97.34% of test samples were correctly predicted, 2.76% were incorrectly predicted.

As for the results of fall detection, this system was tested over 5 persons; all are males, their age ranges between 22 and 28 years old. Each subject performed an average of 5 hours and 20 minutes, and an average of 56 falls. Table 5 summarizes the testing done with the 5 subjects.

As shown in Table 5, 97.14% of falls were correctly detected; however, the system will be tested more with a robotic system to perform continuously so that the number of tests will be more representative.

Table 5. Testing results for the fall detection part

Subject	Age	Test duration (min)	Number of falls	Correctly detected falls	Non detected Falls	Nb. of false detections
1	22	330	50	48	2	0
2	24	315	60	59	1	0
3	22	290	50	48	2	0
4	23	300	55	53	2	0
5	28	350	65	64	1	0

However, the sub-system has shown two basic delays, the first one is the time delay for the Firebase to receive the readings, and the second one is the time delay for the app notification. The average time delay for the Firebase was 1.3 seconds, and the average time delay for the notification was 1.5 seconds.

4. ADVANCED SYSTEM PROCESSING

As mentioned before, this chapter describes two phases of a bigger project that aims to design and implement a safe monitoring system for prediction and detection of epileptic seizures. The first stage was described in the previous section by showing the basic design of the system. As for the second stage, it aims to present a comparative study between several classification methods in order to achieve epileptic seizure prediction and detection. The same design as the one shown in the previous section will be used, but the ANN will be compared to other classification methods.

Thus, in this section, different classification methods will be proposed in order to choose the best one and proceed with next phases of the project. The five classification methods that have been studied are Decision Trees, Discriminant Analysis, SVM, KNN, and Ensemble Learning. They are studied in terms of accuracy, specificity, sensitivity, precision, false detection rate and F-measure.

For the simulation, the CHB-MIT dataset, already presented in the previous section, will be also used.

4.1. Different Classification Methods

4.1.1. Decision Trees

Decision Trees is a classification method that predicts a response by following the decision in a tree from a root node down to a leaf node. For nominal response, like positive or negative, true or false, Decision trees method is suitable. However, for numeric response, Regression Trees method is suitable [90]

When the decision tree is used for classification, the importance of the split is evaluated by either an impurity measure of using the node error. If all the training instances, after a split, are belonging to the same class, the node is pure. However, the probability of a class can be evaluated using different methods. When N_m training instances reach a node m, these instances can be divided into the different classes, so N_m^i is the number of instances at node m that belong to class C_i. Thus, the probability of class C_i at node m is $p_m^i = \frac{N_m^i}{N_m}$. If this probability is 1, then no need for more splits, and a leaf is added with label C_i (the corresponding class) [91].

In order to measure the impurity of a node, different methods can be used as Entropy, Misclassification error and Gini's diversity index. This latter has been use in this study. The Gini's diversity index is given by $1 - \sum_i p^2(i)$ where i is the number of classes at the node, and p(i) is the probability of class i at the node. If the node is pure, then the Gini's index is 0; otherwise it is positive [91].

Table 6. Patient 1 - Decision Tree Learning

Classifier Preset	Prediction Speed (obs/sec)	Training Time (sec)	Max number of splits	Split Criterion	Accuracy (%)	True positive rate (%)		
						i	n	p
Complex Tree	~550	14.27	100	Gini's diversity index	85.2	97	85	62
Medium Tree	~600	12.581	20		85.2	97	85	62
Simple Tree	~470	14.439	4		88.0	93	90	74

A sample case (for patient 1 in Table 5) is shown in Table 6. Three classifier presets – complex tree, medium tree and simple tree - have been used with a maximum number of splits equal to 100, 20 and 4 respectively. The table shows the accuracy and the true positive rate for the three presets with respect to i (ictal state), n (normal state) and p (preictal state).

4.1.2. Discriminant Analysis

Discriminant Analysis is a classification method that predicts responses using different Gaussian distributions; the fitting function calculates the values of Gaussian distribution for the different classes in order to train the classifier. Then, the trained classifier predicts the response by finding the smallest misclassification cost of each class [92].

In discriminant analysis, the data from each class is assumed to have a Gaussian Mixture Distribution. Two models in discriminant analysis are well-known models, the linear discriminant and the quadratic discriminant. In the first, the model has the same covariance matrix for each class, but with different means. The model first calculates the sample mean of each class. As for the calculation of the sample covariance, it subtracts the sample mean from the observations of the class to finally take the empirical covariance matrix of the result. However, in quadratic discriminant, the covariance matrix and the means vary for each class. After calculating the sample mean and covariance, the model takes the empirical covariance matrix of each class [91].

Weighted Classifiers are created for the different classes. M is an N-by-K observations matrix, where K is the number of classes (3 for prediction system and 2 for detection system), and N is the number of observations. $M_{ni} = 1$ if observation n belongs to class C_i, and it is 0 otherwise. So, to calculate the mean of the class, the natural generalization is given by $\widehat{\mu_k} = \frac{\sum_{n=1}^{N} M_{nk} w_n x_n}{\sum_{n=1}^{N} M_{nk} w_k}$ where w_n are the weights, and the unbiased estimate of the pooled-in covariance matrix is given by $\hat{\Sigma} = \frac{\sum_{n=1}^{N} \sum_{k=1}^{K} M_{nk}(x_n - \widehat{\mu_k})(x_n - \widehat{\mu_k})^T}{1 - \sum_{k=1}^{K} \frac{w_k^2}{W_k}}$, where w_k is the sum of the weights for class k *[92]*.

A sample case (for patient 1 in Table 5) is shown in Table 7. The table shows the accuracy and the true positive rate for Discriminant Learning with Linear Discriminant and Quadratic Discriminant Classifier Presets, Diagonal Covariance has been used for regularization.

Table 7. Patient 1 - Discriminant Learning

Discriminant Classifier Preset	Prediction Speed (obs/sec)	Training Time (sec)	Regularization	Accuracy (%)	True positive rate (%)		
					i	n	p
Linear	~320	16.03	Diagonal Covariance	73.1	82	100	0
Quadratic	~330	19.184		86.6	94	91	62

4.1.3. Support Vector Machine

Support Vector Machine (SVM) is a classification and regression method that has been defined by Vapnik and his colleagues in 1995. It relies on kernel functions; thus it is considered nonparametric. The training examples are represented as points in space and mapped in a way that the separate categories are divided by gaps. Then, the same space is used for the testing examples, which are mapped and to be classified based on the gap they fall in *[93]*.

SVM has been originally created for classification problems that have two outputs (2 classes), and especially when data is linearly separable. The objective of SVM is to find the best hyperplane that separates the classes with the largest margin between them. This hyperplane results in two support vectors that are formed using the closest samples from each class to the hyperplane. When data is not linearly separable, the support vectors can be found using a soft margin or a hyperplane that separates most of the data points, but not all of them *[94] [95]*.

In epilepsy system, SVM is challenging due to two main problems: multidimensionality of the data and multiclass (non binary) output (in the 3 classes system for prediction). To overcome the problem of multiclass output, two topologies can be applied: "One vs. the rest" for 3 classes, where 3 binary classifiers are trained to determine whether a data point or sample belongs to its corresponding class or to any of the other classes. As for the second topology, it is "One vs. one" where a binary classifier is trained for each pair of classes, and a voting method is applied later on to combine the outputs.

To overcome the multidimensionality problem, multiclass SVM is created, the data consists of $(x_1^l, l_1), \ldots, (x_N^l, l_N)$, where l is the number of features, N is the number of samples in the dataset, $x_i^l \in \mathbb{R}^L$ representing the features vector, and $l_j \in \{1,2,3\}$ representing the classes. For each class k, in order to separate its corresponding training vectors from the other classes, the kth function $w_k^T \emptyset(x_i^l) + b_k$ is calculated where the optimization is done by solving the minimization equation:

$$\min_{w, b, \zeta} \frac{1}{2}\sum_{k=1}^{3} w_k^T w_k + C \sum_{j=1}^{N} \sum_{k \neq l_j} \zeta_j^k \qquad (1)$$

Subject to: $w_{l_j}^T \phi(x_i^l) + b_{l_j} \geq w_k^T \phi(x_i^l) + b_k + 2 - \zeta_j^k$

Subject to: $\zeta_j^k \geq 0, \quad 1 \leq j \leq= N, \quad k \in \{1,2,3\}\backslash l_j$

The term C is to penalize the training error, b is the bias vector and ξ is the slack variable vector, and Ø is a function to map the deformation vectors to a higher dimensional space. A kernel function K is used to represent similarity between elements of the input space x [93, 96]. Four kernel functions have been investigated in our study:

Linear: $K(x_i, x_j) = \emptyset(x_i)^T \emptyset(x_j) = x_i^T x_j$, (2)

Quadratic: $K(x_i, x_j) = \emptyset(x_i)^T \emptyset(x_j) = (x_i^T x_j + C)^2$, (3)

Cubic: $K(x_i, x_j) = \emptyset(x_i)^T \emptyset(x_j) = (x_i^T x_j + C)^3$, (4)

Gaussian: $K(x_i, x_j) = \emptyset(x_i)^T \emptyset(x_j) = e^{-\gamma(x_i - x_j)^T (x_i - x_j)}$, (5)

γ being the spread of the Gaussian cluster.

A sample case (for patient 1 in Table 5) is shown in Table 8. The table shows the accuracy and the true positive rate for six SVM classification presets: Linear SVM, Quadratic SVM, Cubic SVM, Fine Gaussian SVM, Medium Gaussian SVM and Coarse Gaussian SVM.

Table 8. Patient 1 - Support Vector Machine

Classifier Preset	Prediction Speed (obs/sec)	Training Time (sec)	Kernel Function	Accuracy (%)	True positive rate (%)		
					i	N	p
Linear SVM	~290	11.279	Linear	80.1	95	95	17
Quadratic SVM	~290	15.939	Quadratic	86.6	93	92	62
Cubic SVM	~270	20.285	Cubic	76.9	94	75	45
Fine Gaussian SVM	~280	22.149	Gaussian	83.3	97	97	29
Medium Gaussian SVM	~380	24.968	Gaussian	78.2	97	98	0
Coarse Gaussian SVM	~400	25.716	Gaussian	73.1	82	100	0

4.1.4. K-Nearest Neighbor

K-Nearest Neighbor (KNN) is a classification method that uses distance between points in testing set to points in the training set. It categorizes the points by using various metrics to determine the distance, and among the distance metrics we list Euclidean, Cosine and Minkowski (cubic). To calculate the distance for n dimensional vectors, different metrics can be used. Thus, three distance metrics are investigated in our study. They are shown below along with their equations:

$$\text{Euclidian: } d(x, y) = \sqrt{\sum_{i=1}^{n}(x_i - y_i)^2}, \tag{6}$$

$$\text{Minkowski (cubic): } d(x, y) = \sqrt[3]{\sum_{i=1}^{n}(x_i - y_i)^3}, \tag{7}$$

$$\text{and Cosine: } d(x, y) = \frac{\sum_{i=1}^{n} x_i y_i}{\sum_{i=1}^{n} x_i^2 \sum_{i=1}^{n} y_i^2}. \tag{8}$$

A sample case (for patient 1 in Table 5) is shown in Table 9. The table shows the accuracy and the true positive rate for KNN with the following classifier presets: Fine KNN, Medium KNN, Coarse KNN, Cosine KNN, Cubic KNN and Weighted KNN.

Table 9. Patient 1- K-Nearest Neighbor (KNN)

Classifier Preset	Prediction Speed (obs/sec)	Training Time (sec)	Number of Neighbors	Distance metric	Accuracy (%)	True positive rate (%)		
						i	n	p
Fine KNN	~510	26.301	1	Euclidean	82.4	95	82	57
Medium KNN	~430	28.142	10	Euclidean	81.5	95	98	19
Coarse KNN	~430	28.531	100		72.2	79	100	0
Cosine KNN	~480	29.547	10	Cosine	86.1	95	99	40
Cubic KNN	~500	30.46	10	Minkowski (cubic)	80.6	94	95	21
Weighted KNN	~540	31.868	10	Euclidean	83.8	95	97	33

4.1.5. Ensemble Learning

Ensemble learning is a classification method that combines multiple classification techniques for prediction. It is mainly used to improve the classification/prediction performance of the model, to optimize the features selection and to eliminate the unwanted likelihood selections [97].

A sample case (for patient 1 in Table 5) is shown in Table 10. Five classifier presets have been studied: Boosted Trees, Bagged Tress, Subspace Discriminant, Subspace KNN and RUSBoosted Tress.

- Boosting trees is training multiple learners successively in order to decrease the net error and adjust the weights of decision trees at the end of the training phase;
- Bagging trees consists of creating several subsets of the data and using these subsets to create several decision trees, the average of the different decisions is used at the end to minimize the variance of the decision tree;
- Subspace Discriminant and Subspace KNN ensemble methods use subspaces from the original dataset in order to create several

trainers. Then, the majority-voting method is used to create the ensemble model;
- RUSBoosted Trees (Random Under Sampling Boosted Trees) focuses mainly on balancing the data distribution between the classes by randomly sampling the data;

Table 10. Patient 1- Ensemble Learning

Classifier Preset	Prediction Speed (obs/sec)	Training Time (sec)	Ensemble Method	Learner Type	Accuracy (%)	True positive rate (%)		
						i	n	p
Boosted Trees	~990	33.294	AdaBoost	Decision Tree	35.6	70	17	2
Bagged Tress	~85	56.428	Bag	Decision Tree	89.8	98	92	69
Subspace Discriminant	~61	62.502	Subspace	Discriminant	75.5	90	98	0
Subspace KNN	~38	83.175		Nearest Neighbors	77.3	97	80	31
RUSBoosted Tress	~100	88.591	RUSBoost	Decision Tree	88.0	95	87	74

4.2. Results of the AI algorithms Implementation

The sample study, which has been shown in the previous section for patient 1, was repeated for all the patients in CHB-MIT dataset. In order to compare all the classification methods that have been studied, the following measures were calculated: accuracy, sensitivity, precision, specificity, false detection rate and F-measure. 70% of the dataset were used for training, and the rest were used for testing.

When referring to seizure detection study, three classes were taken into consideration: normal, ictal and preictal. However, when considering the seizure prediction, two classes were taken into consideration: ictal and non-ictal.

The results for three classes (normal, ictal and preictal) are shown in Table 11 where the highest accuracy (90.04%), specificity (93.90%), F-Measure (81.31%) and lowest false detection rate (6.1%) are achieved using the Bagged Trees Ensemble Learning, whereas the highest sensitivity (76.91%) and precision (85.52%) are achieved with Quadratic Support Vector Machine.

Table 11. Results for epilepsy prediction

Method	Accuracy	Sensitivity	Precision	Specificity	FDR	F-Measure
CTL	87.53	73.04	82.21	92.59	7.41	76.92
MTL	87.66	74.59	83.14	93.31	6.69	78.38
STL	85.89	71.52	80.71	92.49	7.51	76.22
LDL	73.73	48.19	63.27	86.06	13.94	56.09
QDL	79.05	61.22	74.19	87.75	12.25	65.82
LSVM	87.34	73.30	81.94	93.36	6.64	77.47
QSVM	89.26	76.91	85.52	93.77	6.23	80.64
CSVM	88.99	75.82	84.46	93.60	6.40	79.55
FGSVM	84.40	66.17	75.56	92.10	7.90	71.33
MGSVM	85.89	68.49	78.14	92.90	7.10	74.76
CGSVM	75.77	48.37	63.97	87.85	12.15	61.08
FKNN	85.40	70.26	79.34	91.93	8.07	73.96
MKNN	81.15	64.54	74.57	91.33	8.67	69.54
CKNN	65.42	38.74	53.50	80.80	19.20	57.87
COSKNN	81.78	62.02	72.93	90.71	9.29	67.27
CUBKNN	82.36	63.51	73.77	90.91	9.09	67.90
WKNN	86.67	72.43	79.88	93.03	6.97	75.18
BTENS	51.80	34.71	47.02	63.77	36.23	65.64
BAGTENS	90.04	75.98	82.53	93.90	6.10	81.31
SUBDIS	82.75	60.84	71.94	92.04	7.96	70.51
SUBKNN	84.24	67.76	76.83	91.52	8.48	71.36
RUSB	87.38	74.96	84.93	93.09	6.91	79.33

The results for two classes (ictal and non-ictal) are shown in Table 12 where the highest accuracy (98.04%) and the F-Measure (97.94%) are achieved with Linear Support Vector, the highest sensitivity (98.00%) and specificity (97.90%) are achieved with Fine Gaussian Support Vector Machine, whereas the highest precision (99.56%) and lowest false detection rate (0.41%) are achieved with Subspace Discriminant Ensemble Learning.

Table 12. Results for epilepsy detection

Method	Accuracy	Sensitivity	Precision	Specificity	False Detection Rate	F-measure
CTL	96.94	97.09	95.97	97.06	4.14	96.51
MTL	96.94	97.14	96.56	97.13	3.50	96.83
STL	96.84	97.14	96.39	97.13	3.68	96.75
LDL	87.67	76.73	97.94	81.35	1.59	85.74
QDL	94.13	93.23	94.68	94.02	5.23	93.70
LSVM	98.04	97.23	98.70	97.32	1.32	97.94
QSVM	96.71	95.68	97.46	95.84	2.50	96.54
CSVM	95.68	94.55	96.63	94.69	3.45	95.52
FGSVM	95.66	98.00	93.50	97.90	7.05	95.64
MGSVM	96.30	94.91	97.43	95.15	2.55	96.09
CGSVM	89.10	83.09	95.65	85.32	6.45	87.97
FKNN	96.91	93.36	95.60	94.34	3.23	93.74
MKNN	94.78	94.09	95.42	94.20	4.95	94.62
CKNN	69.69	66.23	81.86	58.30	28.32	68.83
COSKNN	93.69	90.23	96.81	91.07	3.00	93.32
CUBKNN	94.45	93.73	95.11	93.87	5.27	94.27
WKNN	96.45	95.59	97.05	95.70	3.00	96.28
BTENS	41.37	68.68	43.08	27.25	87.68	52.62
BAGTENS	97.40	97.50	97.11	97.50	2.91	97.30
SUBDIS	95.09	90.45	99.56	91.45	0.41	94.71
SUBKNN	95.64	96.27	94.84	96.25	5.36	95.51
RUSB	44.31	69.27	46.17	35.71	81.05	54.95

Unfortunately, CHB-MIT dataset includes only one sample for ECG recordings (Patient 4), the complete analysis has been repeated after adding the 2 ECG features, the average heart rate per minute and the mean R-R interval distance.

Results are shown in Table 13 where the accuracy and sensitivity for 3 classes (normal, ictal and preictal) and 2 classes (ictal, non-ictal) with and without ECG features for the same patient.

As shown in Table 13, the accuracy and the sensitivity have increased by 1 to 1.8% after adding the ECG features.

Table 13. Patient 4 – Results with and without ECG Features

Method	3 classes				2 classes			
	Accuracy		Sensitivity		Accuracy		Sensitivity	
	No ECG	ECG	No ECG	ECG	No ECG	ECG	No ECG	ECG
CTL	95.30	96.44	90.01	91.36	96.94	98.30	97.09	98.06
MTL	95.30	96.44	90.01	91.45	96.94	98.10	97.14	98.40
STL	95.30	96.44	90.01	91.63	96.84	98.29	97.14	98.79
LDL	82.00	83.48	48.14	49.01	87.67	88.72	76.73	78.11
QDL	89.50	90.40	77.62	78.47	94.13	95.82	93.23	94.72
LSVM	86.60	87.99	70.03	71.15	98.04	99.61	97.23	98.39
QSVM	89.00	90.51	74.85	75.97	96.71	98.45	95.68	96.73
CSVM	88.40	89.73	74.08	75.26	95.68	96.73	94.55	95.77
FSVM	89.00	90.16	81.13	82.19	95.66	97.00	98.00	99.57
MGSVM	84.90	86.00	49.59	50.34	96.30	97.84	94.91	96.62
CGSVM	82.60	83.43	48.38	49.06	89.10	90.34	83.09	84.25
FKNN	94.20	95.80	90.81	92.45	96.91	98.46	93.36	94.76
MKNN	84.90	86.00	49.59	50.49	94.78	96.01	94.09	95.03
CKNN	76.20	77.50	44.90	45.48	69.69	70.39	66.23	67.15
COSKNN	86.00	87.20	66.04	66.97	93.69	95.19	90.23	91.22
CUBKNN	84.30	85.14	49.35	49.89	94.45	95.49	93.73	94.95
WKNN	90.70	91.70	82.60	84.01	96.45	97.80	95.59	96.93
BTENS	41.90	42.44	16.58	16.83	41.37	41.95	68.68	69.51
BAGTENS	95.30	96.54	90.01	91.27	97.40	98.38	97.50	99.26
SUBDIS	82.60	83.67	48.38	49.20	95.09	96.61	90.45	91.45
SUBKNN	91.90	93.46	83.99	85.17	95.64	97.27	96.27	98.01
RUSB	95.30	96.35	88.77	90.10	44.31	45.02	69.27	70.24

CONCLUSION AND FUTURE WORK

The proposed system has been successfully implemented. The accuracy and the resulting mean square error (mse) are acceptable for the first prototype that uses Arduino and Raspberry pi for analog to digital conversion and for signal processing. EEG sensor, ECG sensor and accelerometers were embedded in a wearable overall that suits industrial workplaces. ANN was implemented for detection and prediction of the three epileptic states; normal, preictal and ictal. Best training mse was achieved after using time domain and frequency features with Levenberg-Marquardt optimization, and the best test mse was achieved with the system to allow the monitoring system correctly predict 97.34% of the testing dataset. The fall detection subsystem has achieved an accuracy of 99.89%.

In the second stage, a comparative study for classification methods to predict and detect epilepsy seizures has been presented. Time domain and frequency domain features from EEG and ECG data have been extracted from CHB-MIT Epilepsy Dataset. Five main classification methods have been studied, including Decision Trees, Discriminant Analysis, SVM, KNN and Ensemble Learning. The accuracy, the sensitivity, the precision, the specificity, the false detection rate and the F-Measure have been calculated in order to compare the different methods. The study has been performed for three classes system (ictal, preictlal and normal) and two classes system (ictal and non-ictal). For the three classes study, with only EEG features, the results show that the highest accuracy, specificity and F-Measure, and lowest false detection rate were achieved with Bagged Trees Ensemble Learning. However, the highest sensitivity and precision were achieved with Quadratic Support Vector Machine. For the two classes study, the results show that the highest accuracy and F-Measure were achieved with Linear Support Vector, the highest sensitivity and specificity were achieved with Fine Gaussian Support Vector Machine. The highest precision and lowest false detection rate were achieved with Subspace Discriminant Ensemble Learning. After adding the ECG features, the accuracy and sensitivity have shown an increase.

As previously mentioned, this book chapter presents two stages in a bigger project. The next step will be applying the classification methods to a safety-related microcontroller and evaluating the overall safety of the project after combining the different subsystems, EEG, ECG and Fall Detection. Safety will be evaluated by finding the achievable Safety Integrity Level of the system, where the safety lifecycle will be presented, as well as the Process Hazard Analysis and Layer of Protection Analysis, which will make the system a safety related application applied to biomedical system. The system will be optimized to be comfortable for the patient as well as safe and reliable. In addition, the performance of the final product (full overall with wearable sensors) will be studied.

REFERENCES

[1] Pietrangelo, A. "*HealthLine: Everything You Need to Know About Epilepsy*," 9 January 2017. [Online]. Available: https://www.healthline.com/health/epilepsy. [Accessed 15 August 2019].

[2] "*Epilepsy A public health imperative, WHO's first Global Epilepsy,*" WHO World Health Organization, 2019.

[3] "*Epilepsy Foundation Annual Report FY17*," Epilepsy Foundation, 2017.

[4] Patterson, A., B. Mudigoudar, S. Fulton, A. McGregor, K. Poppel, M. Wheless, L. Brooks and J. Wheless, "SmartWatch by SmartMonitor: Assessment of Seizure Detection Efficacy for Various Seizure Types in Children, a Large Prospective Single-Center Study," *Pediatric Neurology,* vol. 53, no. 4, pp. 309-311, 2015.

[5] Eftekhar, A., W. Juffali, J. El-Emad, T. Constandinou and C. Toumazou, "Ngram-Derived Pattern Recognition for the Detection and Prediction of Epileptic Seizures," *Plos One,* vol. 9, 2014.

[6] VUMC Reporter, Vanderbilt University Medical Center, Department of Neurological Surgery, "Laser Technology Offers New Option to Treat Epilepsy," Vanderbilt University Medical Center, 2015.

[7] Prajacta, H., "Moved By Her Son's Suffering, Mother Invents AI-Powered Glove That Predicts Epileptic Seizures," *Analytics India Magazine,* 30 November 2017.

[8] Sorensen, T., L. Ulrich and I. Conradsen, "Automatic epileptic seizure onset detection using Matching Pursuit: A case study," *Engineering in Medicine and Biology Society (EMBC),* 2010.

[9] Kharbouch, A., A. Shoeb, J. Guttag and S. Cash, "An algorithm for seizure onset detection using intracranial EEG," *Epilepsy Behav,* no. 22, pp. 29-35, 2011.

[10] Acharya, U., S. Sree and J. Suri, "Automatic Detection of Epileptic EEG Signals Using Higher Order Cumulant Features," *International Journal of Neural Systems,* 2011.

[11] Liu, Y., W. Zhou, Q. Yuan and S. Chen, "Automatic seizure detection using wavelet transform and SVM in long-term intracranial EEG," *IEEE Transactions on Neural Systems and Rehabilitation Engineering,* vol. 20, no. 6, pp. 749-755, 2012.

[12] Yuanfa, W., L. Zunchao, F. Lichen, Z. Chuang and Z. Wenhao, ""Automatic Detection of Epilepsy and Seizure Using Multiclass Sparse Extreme Learning Machine Classification," *Computational and Mathematical Methods in Medicine,* 2017.

[13] Petersen, E., J. Dunn-Henriksen, A. Amzaretto, T. Kjaer, C. Thomsen and H. Sorensen, "Generic single- channel detection of absence seizures," in *Engineering in Medicine and Biology Society (EMBC),* Boston, 2011.

[14] Golshan Taheri, B., Y. Mehran, K. Alireza and R. Arash, "Detection of Epileptic Seizure Using Wireless Sensor Networks," *Journal of Medical Signals and Sensors,* pp. 63-68, 2013.

[15] Wang, L., X. Weining, L. Yang, L. Meilin, H. Jie, C. Weigang and H. Chao, "Automatic Epileptic Seizure Detection in EEG Signals Using Multi-Domain Feature Extraction and Nonlinear Analysis," *Entropy,* vol. 19, no. 6, 2019.

[16] Chisci, L., A. Mavino, G. Perferi, M. Sciandrone, C. Anile, G. Colicchio and Fugettaf., "RealTime Epileptic Seizure Prediction Using AR Models and Support Vector Machines," *IEEE Transactions on Biomedical Engineering,* vol. 57, no. 5, 2010.

[17] Teixeira, C., G. Favaro, B. Direito, M. Bandarabadi, H. Feldwisch-Drentrup, M. Ihle, C. Alvarado, Q. Le Van, M. Bjorn Schelter, A. Schulze-Bonhage, F. Sales, V. Navarro and D. Dourado, "Brainatic: A System for Real-Time Epileptic Seizure Prediction," in *Biosystems & Biorobotics,* 2014, pp. 7-17.

[18] Parvez M. and M. Paul, ""EEG Signal Classification using Frequency Band Analysis towards Epileptic Seizure Prediction",," in *16th Int'l Conf. Computer and Information Technology,* Khulna, Bangladesh, 2014.

[19] Maiwald, T., M. Winterhalder, R. Aschenbrenner-Scheibe, H. Voss, A. Schulze-Bonhage and J. Timmer, "Comparison of three nonlinear

seizure prediction methods by means of the seizure prediction characteristic," *Physical D: Nonlinear Phenomena,* vol. 194, no. 3-4, pp. 357-368, 2004.

[20] Winterhalder, M., B. Schelter, T. Maiwald, A. Brandt, A. Schad, A. Schulze-Bonhage and J. Timmer, "Spatio-temporal patient–individual assessment of synchronization changes for epileptic seizure prediction," *Clinical Neurophysiology,* vol. 117, no. 11, pp. 2399-2413, 2006.

[21] Park, Y., L. Luo, K. Parhi and T. Netoff, ""Seizure prediction with spectral power of EEG using cost-sensitive support vector machines," *Epilepsia,* vol. 52, no. 10, pp. 1761-1770, 2011.

[22] Gadhoumi, K., J. Lina and J. Gotman, ""Discriminating preictal and interictal states in patients with temporal lobe epilepsy using wavelet analysis of intracerebral EEG," *Clinical Neurophysiology,* vol. 123, no. 10, pp. 1906-1916, 2012.

[23] Li, S., W. Zhou, Q. Yuan and Y. Liu, "Seizure prediction using spike rate of intracranial EEG," *IEEE Transactions on Neural Systems and Rehabilitation Engineering,* vol. 21, no. 6, pp. 880-886, 2013.

[24] Zheng, Y., G. Wang, K. Li, G. Bao and J. Wang, ""Epileptic seizure prediction using phase synchronization based on bivariate empirical mode decomposition," *Clinical Neurophysiology,* vol. 125, no. 6, pp. 1104-1111, 2014.

[25] Aarabi, A. and B. He, "Seizure prediction in hippocampal and neocortical epilepsy using a model-based approach," *Clinical Neurophysiology,* vol. 125, no. 5, pp. 930-940, 2014.

[26] Zhang, Z. and K. Parhi, "Low-complexity seizure prediction from iEEG/sEEG using spectral power and ratios of spectral power," *IEEE Transactions on Biomedical Circuits and Systems,* vol. 10, no. 3, pp. 693-706, 2016.

[27] Parvez, M. and M. Paul, "Seizure prediction using undulated global and local features," *IEEE Transactions on Biomedical Engineering,* vol. 64, no. 1, pp. 208-2017, 2017.

[28] Sharif, B. and A. Jafari, "Prediction of epileptic seizures from EEG using analysis of ictal rules on Poincaré plane," *Computer Methods and Programs in Biomedicine,* vol. 145, pp. 11-22, 2017.

[29] Aarabi A. and B. He., "Seizure prediction in patients with focal hippocampal epilepsy," *Clinical Neurophysiology,* vol. 128, no. 7, pp. 1299-1307, 2017.

[30] Goldberger, A., L. Amaral, L. Glass, J. Hausdorff, P. Ivanov, R. Mark, J. Mietus, G. Moody, C. Peng, H. Stanley, PhysioBank, PhysioToolkit and PhysioNet, "Components of a New Research Resource for Complex Physiologic Signals," *Circulation,* vol. 101, no. 23, pp. e2015-e220, 2000.

[31] Shoeb, A., *"Application of Machine Learning to Epileptic Seizure Onset Detection and Treatment,"* Ph.D. thesis, Massachusetts Institute of Technology, 2009.

[32] Zabihi, M., S. Kiranyaz, A. Rad, A. Katsaggelos, M. Gabbouj and T. Ince, "Analysis of high-Dimensional phase space via poincare section for patient-Specific seizure detection," *IEEE Transactions on Neural Systems and Rehabilitation Engineering,* vol. 24, no. 3, pp. 386-398, 2016.

[33] Hills, M., " Seizure Detection Using FFT, Temporal and Spectral Correlation Coefficients, Eigenvalues and Random Forest," Technical Report, Github, 2014.

[34] Fergus, P., A. Hussain, D. Hingett, D. Al-Jumeily, K. Abdel-Aziz and H. Hamdan, " A machine learning system for automated whole-brain seizure detection," *Applied Computing and Informatics,* vol. 12, no. 1, pp. 70-89, 2016.

[35] Xan, G., X. Jia and A. Zhang, "Context-learning based electroencephalogram analysis for epileptic seizure detection," *IEEE International Conference on Bioinformatics and Biomedicine (BIBM),* pp. 325-330, 2015.

[36] Chen, D., S. Wan, J. Xiang and F. Bao, "A high-performance seizure detection algorithm based on Discrete Wavelet Transform (DWT) and EEG," *PLoS ONE,* vol. 12, no. 3, 2017.

[37] Siddharth, P., P. Adam, M. Tinoosh and O. Tim, " Detecting Epileptic Seizures from EEG Data using Neural Networks," 2014. [Online]. Available: https://arxiv.org/abs/1412.6502.

[38] Turner, J., P. Adam, M. Tinoosh and O. Tim, " Deep belief networks used on high resolution multichannel electroencephalography data for seizure detection," AAAI Spring Symposium Series, 2014.

[39] Ye, Y., X. Guangxu, J. Kebin and Z. Aidong, "A Multi- view Deep Learning Method for Epileptic Seizure Detection using Short- time Fourier Transform," in *8th ACM International Conference on Bioinformatics, Computational Biology,and Health Informatics (ACM-BCB '17)*, New York, USA, 2017.

[40] Akara, S., L. Ling and G. Yike, "Feature extraction with stacked autoencoders for epileptic seizure detection," in *36th Annual International Conference in Engineering in Medicine and Biology Society (EMBC)*, Chicago, IL, USA. [, 2014.

[41] Thodoroff, P., J. Pineau and A. Lim, "Learning robust features using deep learning for automatic seizure detection," in *1st Machine Learning for Healthcare Conference*, 2016.

[42] Muhammad, G., M. Masud, S. Amin, R. Alrobaea and M. Alhamid, "Automatic Seizure Detection in a Mobile Multimedia Framework," *IEEE Access,* vol. 6, pp. 45372-45383, 2018.

[43] Vallabh P., and R. Malekian, "Fall detection monitoring systems: a comprehensive review," *Journal of Ambient Intelligence and Humanized Computing,* 2017.

[44] Hakim, A., M. Huq, S. Shanta and B. Ibrahim, " Smartphone based data mining for fall detection: analysis and design," *Procedia computer science,* vol. 105, pp. 46-51, 2017.

[45] R., Gibson, Amira A., N. Ramzan, P. Casaseca-de-la-Higuera and Z. Pervez, "Multiple comparator classifier framework for accelerometer-based fall detection and diagnostic," *Applied Soft Computing,* vol. 39, pp. 94-103, 2016.

[46] Van De Ven, P., H. O'Brien, J. Nelson and A. Clifford, "Unobtrusive monitoring and identification of fall accidents," *Medical engineering & physics,* vol. 37, no. 5, pp. 499-504, 2015.

[47] Shen, V., H. Lai and A. Lai, " The implementation of a smartphone-based fall detection system using a high level fuzzy petri net," *Applied Soft Computing,* vol. 26, pp. 390-400, 2015.

[48] Leone, A., G. Rescio, A. Caroppo and P. Siciliano, "A wearable emg-based system pre-fall detector," *Procedia Engineering,* vol. 120, pp. 455-458, 2015.

[49] Pannurat, N., S. Thiemjarus and E. Nantajeewarawat, " A hybrid temporal reasoning framework for fall monitoring.," *IEEE Sens,* vol. 17, pp. 1749-1759, 2017.

[50] Ozcan, K., S. Velipasalar and P. Varshney, "Autonomous fall detection with wearable cameras by using relative entropy distance measure," *IEEE Transactions on Human-Machine Systems,* vol. 47, no. 1, pp. 31-39, 2017.

[51] Sabatini, A., G. Ligorio, A. Mannini, V. Genovese and L. Pinna, " Prior-to-and post-impact fall detection using inertial and barometric altimeter measurements," *IEEE transactions on neural systems and rehabilitation engineering,* vol. 24, no. 7, pp. 774-783, 2016.

[52] Jian, H. and H. Chen, "A portable fall detection and alerting system based on KNN algorithm and remote medicine," *China Communications,* vol. 12, no. 4, pp. 23-31, 2015.

[53] Kau, L. and C. Chen, " A smart phone-based pocket fall accident detection, positioning, and rescue system," *IEEE journal of biomedical and health informatics,* vol. 19, no. 1, pp. 44-56, 2015.

[54] Wang, J. Z. Zhang, B. Li, S. Lee and R. Sherratt, "An enhanced fall detection system for elderly person monitoring using consumer home networks," *IEEE transactions on consumer electronics,* vol. 60, no. 1, pp. 23-29, 2014.

[55] Karantonis, D., M. Narayanan, M. Mathie, N. Lovell and B. Celler, " Implementation of a real-time human movement classifier using a triaxial accelerometer for ambulatory monitoring," *IEEE transactions on information technology in biomedicine,* vol. 10, no. 1, pp. 156-167, 2006.

[56] Zhang, T., J. Wang, L. Xu and P. Liu, " Fall detection by wearable sensor and one-class svm algorithm.," *Intelligent computing in signal processing and pattern recognition,* pp. 858-863, 2006.

[57] Bourke A., and G. Lyons, "A threshold-based fall detection algorithm using a bi-axial gyroscope sensor," *Medical engineering & physics,* vol. 30, no. 1, pp. 84-90, 2008.

[58] Aniana, G., A. Tognetti, N. Carbonaro, M. Tesconi, F. Cutolo, G. Zupone and D. De Rossi, "Development of a novel algorithm for human fall detection using wearable sensors," *Sensors,* pp. 1336-1339, 2008.

[59] Lai, C., S. Chang, H. Chao and Y. Huang, "Detection of cognitive injured body region using multiple triaxial accelerometers for elderly falling," *IEEE Sensors Journal,* vol. 11, no. 3, pp. 763-770, 2011.

[60] Bianchi, F., S. Redmond, M. Narayanan, Cerutti S. and Lovell N., " Barometric pressure and triaxial accelerometry-based falls event detection," *IEEE Transactions on Neural Systems and Rehabilitation Engineering,* vol. 18, no. 6, pp. 619-627, 2010.

[61] Yazar, A., F. Keskin, B. Torein and A. Cetin, "Fall detection using single-tree complex wavelet transform," *Pattern Recognition Letters,* vol. 34, no. 15, pp. 1945-1952, 2013.

[62] Zigel, Y., D. Litvak and I. Gannot, " A method for automatic fall detection of elderly people using floor vibrations and soundproof of concept on human mimicking doll falls," *IEEE Transactions on Biomedical Engineering,* vol. 56, no. 12, pp. 2858-2867, 2009.

[63] Li, Y., K. Ho and M. Popescu, "A microphone array system for automatic fall detection," *IEEE Transactions on Biomedical Engineering,* vol. 59, no. 5, pp. 1291-1301, 2012.

[64] Liu, L., M. Popescu, M. Skubic and M. Rantz, "An automatic fall detection framework using data fusion of doppler radar and motion sensor network," in *Engineering in Medicine and Biology Society (EMBC)*, 2014.

[65] Litvak, D., Zigel Y. and Gannoti., "Fall detection of elderly through floor vibrations and sound," in *Engineering in Medicine and Biology Society*, 2008.

[66] Khan, M., M. Yu, P. Feng, L. Wang and J. Chambers, "An unsupervised acoustic fall detection system using source separation for sound interference suppression," *Signal processing,* vol. 110, pp. 199-210, 2015.

[67] Alwan, M., P. Rajendran, S. Kell, D. Mack, S. Dalal, M. Wolfe and R. Felder, "A smart and passive floor-vibration based fall detector for elderly," *Information and Communication Technologies,* vol. 1, no. 2, pp. 1003-1007, 2006.

[68] Zhuang, X., J. Huang, G. Potamianos and M. Hasegawa-Johnson, "Acoustic fall detection using Gaussian mixture models and gmm supervectors," in *International Conference On Acoustics, Speech and Signal Processing ICASSP,* 2009.

[69] Werner, F., J. Diermaier, S. Schmid and P. Panek, "Fall detection with distributed floor-mounted accelerometers, An overview of the development and evaluation of a fall detection system," in *Pervasive Computing Technologies for Healthcare (PervasiveHealth),* 2011.

[70] Chaccour, K., R. Darazi, A. El Hassan and E. Andres, "Smart carpet using differential piezoresistive pressure sensors for elderly fall detection," in *Wireless and Mobile Computing, Networking and Communications (WiMob),* 2015.

[71] Popescu, M., B. Hotrabhavananda, M. Moore and M. Skubic, "Vampir - an automatic fall detection system using a vertical PIR sensor array," in *Pervasive Computing Technologies for Healthcare (PervasiveHealth),* 2012.

[72] Tomii S. and T. Ohtsuki, "Falling detection using multiple doppler sensors. In: e-Health Networking," in *Applications and Services (Healthcom),* 2012.

[73] Rimminen, H., J. Lindstrom, M. Linnavuo and R. Sepponen, "Detection of falls among the elderly by a floor sensor using the electric near field," *IEEE Transactions on Information Technology in Biomedicine,* vol. 14, no. 6, pp. 1475-1476, 2010.

[74] Nizam Y. and I. Gu, "Human fall detection from depth images using position and velocity of subject," *Procedia Computer Science,* vol. 105, pp. 131-137, 2017.

[75] Yun Y.and I. Gu., " Human fall detection in videos by fusing statistical features of shape and motion dynamics on riemannian manifolds," *Neurocomputing,* vol. 207, pp. 726-734, 2016.

[76] Kwolek B. and M. Kepski, "Fuzzy inference-based fall detection using Kinect and body-worn accelerometer," *Applied Soft Computing,* vol. 40, pp. 305-318, 2016.

[77] Yang S. and S. Lin, "Fall detection for multiple pedestrians using depth image processing technique," *Computer methods and programs in biomedicine,* vol. 114, no. 2, pp. 172-182, 2014.

[78] Kolek B., and M. Kepski, " Human fall detection on embedded platform using depth maps and wireless accelerometer," *Computer methods and programs in biomedicine,* vol. 117, no. 3, pp. 489-501, 2014.

[79] Bosch B.,and M. Kepski, " Fall detection based on the gravity vector using a wide-angle camera," *Expert Systems with Applications,* vol. 41, no. 17, pp. 7980-7986, 2014.

[80] Rougier, C., E. Auvinet, J. Rousseau and J. Meunier, "Fall detection from depth map video sequences," *International Conference on Smart Homes and Health Telematics,* p. 121128, 2011.

[81] Auvinet, E., F. Multon, A. Saint-Arnaud and J. Rousseau, " Fall detection with multiple cameras: An occlusion-resistant method based on 3-d silhouette vertical distribution," *Transactions on Information Technology in Biomedicine,* vol. 15, no. 2, pp. 290-300, 2011.

[82] Rougier, C., J. Meunier, A. St-Arnaud, J. Rousseau and J. Meunier, " Fall detection from human shape and motion history using video surveillance," *Advanced Information Networking and Applications Workshops,* vol. 2, pp. 875-880, 2017.

[83] Yu, M., Y. Yu, A. Rhuma, S. Naqvi, L. Wang and J. Chambers, "An online one class support vector machine-based person-specific fall detection system for monitoring an elderly individual in a room environment," *IEEE journal of biomedical and health informatics,* vol. 2, pp. 875-880, 2013.

[84] Rougier, C., J. Meunier, A. St-Arnaud and J. Rousseau, "Monocular 3d head tracking to detect falls of elderly people," *Engineering in Medicine and Biology Society,* pp. 6384-6387, 2006.

[85] Hazelhoff, L., J. Han and H. Peter, "Video-based fall detection in the home using principal component analysis," in *International Conference on Advanced Concepts for Intelligent Vision Systems,* 2008.

[86] Faroughi, H., A. Rezvanian and A. Paziraee, "Robust fall detection using human shape and multiclass support vector machine," in *Computer Vision, Graphics & Image Processing,* 2008.

[87] Hsu, Y., J. Hsieh, H. Kao and H. Liao, "Human behavior analysis using deformable triangulations," in *Multimedia Signal Processing,* 2005.

[88] Krekovic, M., P. Ceric, T. Dominko, M. Ilijas, K. Ivancic, V. Skolan and J. Sarlija, "A method for real-time detection of human fall from video," in *Proceedings of the 35th International Convention,* 2012.

[89] Haykin, S. Neural Networks: A Comprehensive Foundation, Delhi, India: Pearson Prentice Hall, 2005.

[90] Breiman, L., J. Friedman, R. Olshen and C. Stone, Classification and Regression Tress, Boca Raton, FL: Chapman & Hall, 1984.

[91] Alaydin, E. Introduction to Machine Learning, Second Edition, Massachusetts London, England: The MIT Press Cambridge, 2010.

[92] Fisher, R. "The Use of Multiple Measurements in Taxonomic Problems," *Annals of Eugenics,* vol. 7, pp. 179-188, 1936.

[93] Vapnik, V. The Nature of Statistical Learning Theory, New York: Springer, 1995.

[94] Hastie, T., R. Tibshirani and J. Friedman, *The Elements of Statistical Learning,* second edition, New York: Springer, 2008.

[95] Christianini, N. and J. Shawe-Taylor, *An Introduction to Support Vector Machines and Other Kernel-Based Learning Methods,* Cambridge, UK: Cambridge University Press, 2000.

[96] Weston, J. and C. Watkins, "Multi-class Support Vec- tor Machines," *Tech. Rep. Technical Report* CSD-TR-98-04, 1998.

[97] Dietterich, T. "Ensemble Methods in Machine Learning," *Int. Workshop on Multiple Classifier Systems, Lecture Notes in Computer Science,* vol. 1857, pp. 1-15, 2000.

In: Vital Signs: An Overview
Editors: Roy Abi Zeid Daou et al.
ISBN: 978-1-53617-765-7
© 2020 Nova Science Publishers, Inc.

Chapter 4

SAFER DRUG ADMINISTRATION VIA SMART SYRINGE PUMP USING PATIENT'S MONITOR FEEDBACK

Hasnaa ElKheshen[1], Ibrahim Deni[1], Alaa Baalbaky[1], Saeed H. Bamashmos[1], Mohamad Dib[2], Lara Hamawy[1], Mohamad Hajj-Hassan[1], Mohamad Abou Ali[1] and Abdallah Kassem[3,*]

[1]Department of Biomedical Engineering,
Lebanese International University, Lebanon
[2]Department of Biomedical Engineering,
Med Consul MEA, Lebanon
[3]ECCE Department, Faculty of Engineering,
Notre Dame University, Lebanon

---

[*] Corresponding Author's Email: akassem@ndu.edu.lb.

ABSTRACT

A stage 2 hypertensive patient is a patient diagnosed with a systolic pressure of 140 mm Hg or higher, or a diastolic pressure of 90 mm Hg or higher. Such patient is a typical example of an intensive care patient, who requires an administration of a high-risk medication via an electric syringe infusion pump. Firstly, a high flow-rate of the drug is entered within a permitted range. Then, a periodic manual decrease of the flow-rate via an intensive care nurse is made based on the patient's blood pressure readings to reach a final patient recovery day. However, an overloaded busy schedule of an intensive care nurse could jeopardize the patient's life due to the improper follow-up of the patient's condition. An automated correlation of a flow-rate of a syringe infusion pump with the patient's blood pressure readings could present a solution for such life-threatening problems. In this paper, an integrated system of a smart syringe pump with a patient monitor's readings capability is proposed to overcome such hazardous problems. Additionally, this allows nurses to save time and focus on other essential duties. Lastly, this work can be considered as an advanced step toward fully automated treatment and monitoring of patients in the intensive care environment.

Keywords: smart syringe pump, automation, microcontroller, calibration, drug library, intelligent ICU, flow rate, physiological patient monitor

INTRODUCTION

Patients, who are under a high-risk medical condition and need special care, are admitted into a specialized hospital department, known as intensive care unit (ICU). This type of unit can be divided into three levels. Level-1 provides the patients with the capabilities of non-invasive monitoring, the oxygen supply, and higher critical nursing care than the one usually provided in a general ward. As for Level-2, it is essentially dedicated for patients with higher demands such as invasive monitoring and basic life support; however, this is only required for a short period. The last level is Level-3; it differs from the previously mentioned levels by providing a complete range of monitoring services and life support technologies [1].

Integrating the Healthcare Enterprise (IHE) is an international non-profit organization. IHE aims to enhance and to share the information of medical devices made by the different manufacturers in a healthcare facility. As a consequence, this leads to simplify the integration of the hospital information system (HIS) in particular the electronic medical record (EMR). To achieve such a goal, the IHE has developed a set of international standards to transfer the clinical as well as administrative data. These standards are known as Healthcare Level-7 (HL7) [2].

Despite this, a major challenge and requirement for the medical staff is the capability to deal with the many medical devices simultaneously. These medical devices usually are made by different manufacturers with different standards and technical requirements. Consequently, there are many different graphical user interfaces (GUI), which the medical staff needs to switch between them. This consumes the healthcare teams' time, who are suffering from a shortage in their numbers. As a result, this jeopardizes the life and safety of the critically ill patients, who are currently being served [3].

In order to simplify the compexity of dealing with many medical devices simultaneously in different situations, and to reduce the nurses' workload, a partially or a fully automation system can be used in such complicated environments. A smart syringe infusion pump is proposed in this paper that can be used in different situations. It uses the feedback of patient's physiological parameters collected from a patient monitor to guide the administration of high-risk medications. Consequently, an integration system between these devices is made. Prior to proceeding in the discussion of the proposed system, a definition of both a patient monitor and a smart syringe infusion pump will be given.

A syringe infusion pump is a medical device, used primarily in miscellaneous nursing departments especially in the intensive care units (neonatal, pediatric and adult) to deliver nourishment or to intravenously administrate drugs in a small precise and an accurate flow rate over a prolonged period of time. An example of the delivery of such drugs is the administration of high-risk medications to control the patient's blood pressure, heart rate, and others. The aim of intravenous drug delivery via the circulatory system is the minimization of the administration's route and time to urgently treat patients with serious health conditions in an effective way. This technique is mainly used in urgent situtations instead of using the oral path as a method of drug delivery because of its inefficiency and slowness. A typical model of a conventional syringe pump is shown in Figure 1.

The use of a syringe infusion pump for the drug's delivery requires the entrance of patient's credentials, the name of the drug, and two parameters: 1- volume and time, 2- flow and time or flow and volume. The third parameter will be calculated automatically by the software.

A smart syringe infusion pump is the recent generation of the syringe infusion pumps, which has many capabilities such as the integration of drug library, barcode scanning, and wireless communication. The proposed system can make the administration of drug safer. It also saves the time of the medical staff.

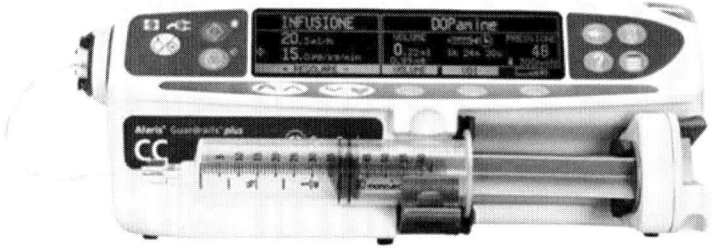

Figure 1. A model of a syringe infusion pump [4].

As for the patient monitor, it becomes currently an indispensable medical device used in the continuous assessment and monitoring of patient's physiological conditions and parameters. This includes the patient's blood pressure (BP either invasively or non-invasively), the electrocardiograph (ECG), the electro-encephalogram (EEG), the non-invasive oxygen blood saturation (SpO_2), the cardiac output (CO), the level of consciousness (also know the bi-spectral index), the temperature, etc. A typical model for a patient monitor is shown in Figure 2.

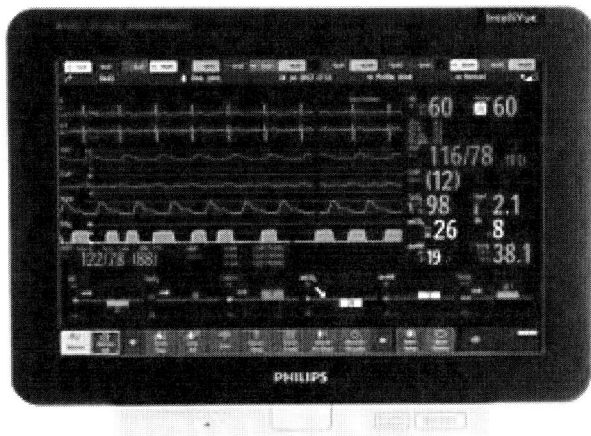

Figure 2. A typical patient monitor [5].

The use of a syringe infusion pump could accidentally lead to the occurrence of some errors made by the operator or the physician. An example of such errors could be either the entrance of the incorrect dose, rate, concentration or even medication [6].

A partial or complete solution and remedy of such errors is the automated communication and control to minimize the risk of seriously ill patients and accordingly the mortality rate.

LITERATURE REVIEW AND SYSTEM OVERVIEW

In the German Heart Center (Berlin), a study was made to explore the advantages of an automated drug administration in the case of critically ill patients. One category of the subjects in this study was post-cardiac surgery patients, who are generally suffering from a cardiovascular instability. Such condition needs the management of infusing miscellaneous vasoactive drugs [7].

A proposal was adopted and made based on the use of the patient's parameters collected via a physiological patient monitor as a feedback to trigger and control the infusion of drugs automatically [7]. Nevertheless, this work was achieved using a MATLAB simulation of a multi-compartmental model.

An additional study was made in the German Heart Center in Munich. This study targeted the test of automation of a heart-lung device [8].

Moreover, similar work and effort was adopted to control the automatic patient's sedation in a critical care unit (CCU) and similarly this was applied in the intraoperative anesthesia [9]. Furthermore, this was used to automatically turn a comatose patient in an ICU bed [10].

System Overview

An automated communication between medical devices in ICU, for example between a syringe pump and a patient monitor, could be one of the next generation biomedical engineering goals. Its results show the importance of using a smart syringe pump with a patient monitor in limiting the number of hemodynamic incidents and in reducing the nursing workload.

Computerized patient infusion devices (called smart pumps or smart infusion pumps) that embrace options for administration's error reduction and knowledge assortment, represent new clinical methods. They can highly reduce the occurrence of intravenous (IV) medication mistakes in hospitals. This technology enables medication error-reduction capabilities through programmed dose limit notifications with audio/visual feedback about wrong dose calculations and programming errors.

The proposed system will automatically correct any error caused by nurses or any medical staff before putting the patient in danger with the availability of further communication with a corresponding physician. The patient monitor will measure the vital signs of the patient non-invasively and the appropriate command will be taken by communicating with the smart syringe pump having a built-in drug library to stop, increase or decrease drug flow automatically.

In addition, proposed system would also work well to enhance patients' care. This especially includes those who, need monitoring and evaluation of their vital signs calculated by a patient monitor. Besides, these patients require an appropriate change in the syringe pump parameters. To accomplish such task, skilled nurses with high qualifications to care for critically ill patients are mandatory.

However, the introduction of this automated system will reduce the large number of nurses specified for monitoring patients in ICU. Eventually, this will decrease human errors, which may sometimes lead to the death of patients.

Requirements and Specification Analysis

To maximize the benefits of the smart pumps and highlight their results on reducing errors and their positive impact on the process of medication administration, several objective systematic reviews of different studies and reports were conducted on systems related to smart pump implementation and its usage.

In the intensive care unit (ICU), medication errors can be considered frequent and may lead to patient morbidity and mortality. In addition, the increased length of ICU stay results in substantial extra cost. Therefore, a system is needed to reduce the incidence and severity of medication administration errors; the study included the importance of introducing a system designed for simultaneous data acquisition from patient monitor and syringe pumps in the intensive care unit system [11].

The success of this proposed system can be considered as a forward step toward a fully automated ICU solution. This includes a situation where any medical device connected to a patient can send or receive a feedback (data) and should be able to easily control specific parameters without affecting any other information.

In addition, a drug library is also being a part of the syringe infusion pump's software that contains information about several drugs including the flow, the volume, the concentration and the rate of infusion. It can help the physician and/or the nurse to select the right parameters of the corresponding drug according to the pre-inserted patients' medical information.

SYSTEM ARCHITECTURE

To implement such system in the ICU of the hospital, a detailed collaboration with physicians and nurses is needed to learn about their treatment approaches. Therefore, a visit to the hospital, especially the ICU, is necessary to identify the system used to monitor the patient and the syringe pumps connected to him or her in order to determine how the proposed system needs to be integrated in the ICU.

The patient's safety should be considered as a high priority when implementing any system such as the proposed one. The workflow of the medical staffs should be respected which makes possible the data collections. This facilitates to provide a specific data that can be used for different purposes. Also, the practice of the physicians can be analyzed and used as training input for automated system. Furthermore, numerous patients' reactions to certain medicines delivered by the syringe pump have been collected from real situations. This collected data is used to enhance the simulation environment [1], which is employed to check the system controllers. Note that, the analysis of the information can offer deeper approaches into common crucial situations, which occur often after a specific operation and/or precondition.

The device is covered by plastic made of PLA Cetus using 3D printer. All the parts of the proposed system were drawn using Fusion360 Autodesk with specific and precise measurements, as shown in Figures 3, 4 and 5.

Figure 3 shows the cover case, where the Nexion LCD 7-inch screen will be installed just above the threaded rod linear guide rail to cover it. In addition, the encoder and servo motor will be installed on the right and left sides of the case.

Figure 4 shows the syringe holder case, where the syringe will be installed connected to a potentiometer that detects its diameter.

The arm connected to the movable part of the linear guide rail is shown in the Figure 5. It is used to push the plunger according to the calculated flow. The circle part contains the limit switch to measure the distance from the start of the linear guide rail to the plunger.

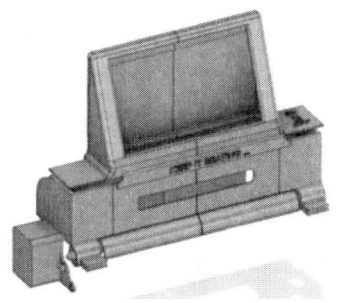

Figure 3. The case of the screen (Fusion 360).

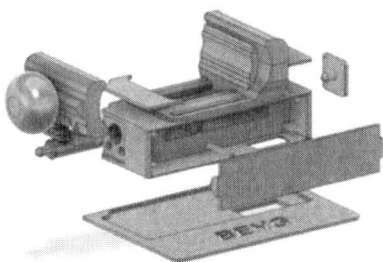

Figure 4. Syringe holder base (Fusion 360).

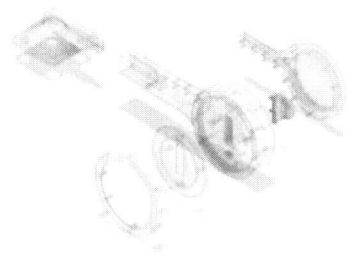

Figure 5. Arm that pushes the syringe's plunger, drawn using Fusion 360.

Components and Modules

Different components and modules were used to realize a prototype of the proposed system. Sensors are used to detect the different parameters taken from the patient's body and display them on a clear touch screen. In addition to the parts related to the syringe pump, the syringe's volume and the movement of the syringe's plunger will be controlled according to a specific needed flow based on the patient's situation.

The next paragraphs will explain the main use of the different component used to realize this prototype.

- ESP-01 module: WiFi Transceiver Module, a helpful way to connect to a WIFI network using a controller system such as Arduino or other microcontrollers. This module does not need a host controller because it runs independently. Sensors and/or peripherals are directly connected to this module. The ESP-01 module is shown in Figure 6.

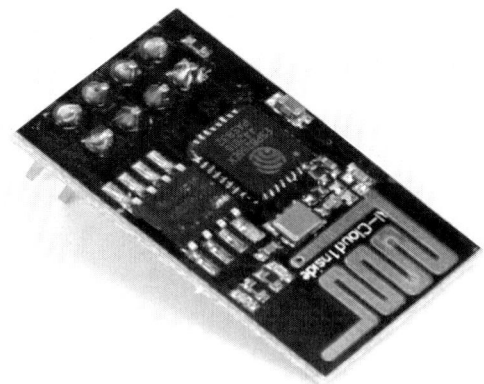

Figure 6. ESP01 WIFI Module.

- AD8232 ECG module: This module, shown in Figure 7, reads the ECG signals from the probes connected to the patient.

Safer Drug Administration via Smart Syringe Pump ...   91

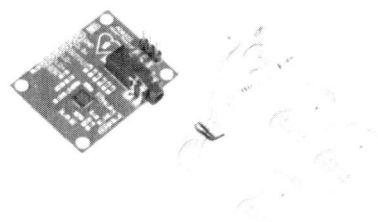

Figure 7. AD8232 ECG module with electrodes.

- DS-100A: Nellcor SpO_2 sensor shown in Figure 8 is used for noninvasive measurement of the patient's oxygen saturation. One side is clipped on the fingertip of the patient and the other side is linked to the patient monitor connected to the main system.

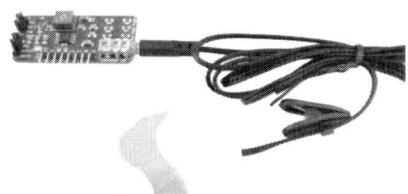

Figure 8. SpO_2 module.

- Easy Pulse: The Pulse Sensor shown in Figure 9 is a heart-beat-rate. It produces a fast and accurate pulse reading due the use of the embedded amplifier with noise removal of the optical heart rate sensor.

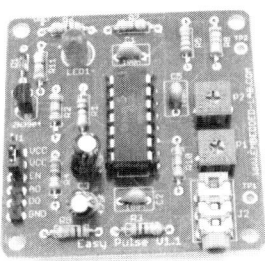

Figure 9. Pulse Sensor Module.

- LM35: The LM35 device, shown in Figure 10, is a temperature sensor with an embedded circuit that enables the detection of temperature in Celsius (Centigrade). It is used to detect the patient's temperature.

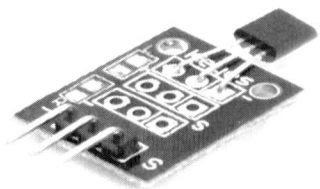

Figure 10. LM35 temperature sensor.

- DHT21: It is a digital humidity and temperature sensor placed on one side of the device. It detects the patient room temperature and humidity. The DHT21 device is shown in Figure 11.

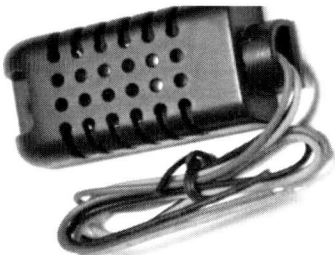

Figure 11. DHT21 sensor.

- DS1302: It is called a Real-time clock. It is used to computes the seconds, minutes, hours and dates which are displayed on the screen. The DS1302 device is shown in Figure 12.

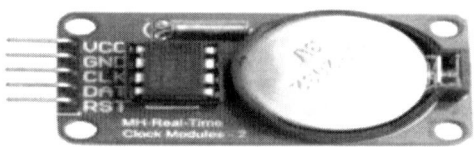

Figure 12. DS1302 real time clock.

- MG995: This is the most famous digital metal gear with high torque servo motor used for the rotation of the threaded rod linear guide rail axis. It is used to push the syringe's arm. Both the servo motor and the linear guide rail are shown in Figure 13.

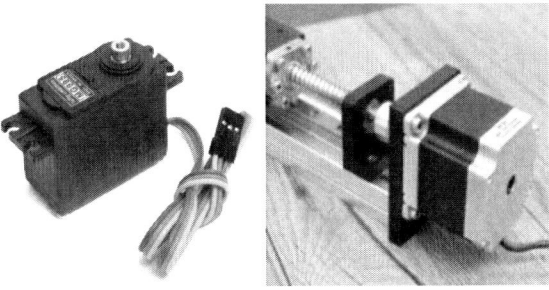

Figure 13. MG995 servo motor and threaded rod linear guide rail.

- Arduino: Figure 14 showed an open-source platform call Arduino. It is the main heart of the prototype. It consists of a physical programmable circuit board (a microcontroller) and a software program.

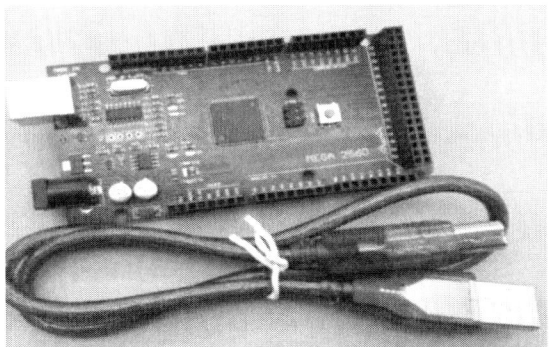

Figure 14. Arduino platform.

- Buzzer RGB Module: The RGB full-color LED Module, shown in Figure 15, is used to mix the red, green and blue colors in order to produce a range of different colors.

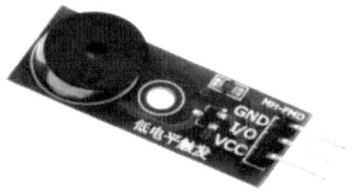

Figure 15. Buzzer RGB module.

- SD Card Module: The SD Card Module is an easy useful way to transfer data to and/or from a standard SD card. The module shown in Figure 16 has SPI interface which is compatible with any SD card.

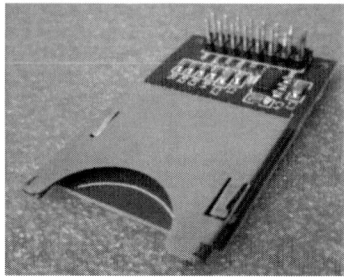

Figure 16. SD Card Module.

- Threaded Rod Linear Guide Rail: It is a robotic arm kit shown in Figure 17 with a motor and a ball screw for CNC. Its linear module is used for the movement of the arm that pushes the syringe's plunger.

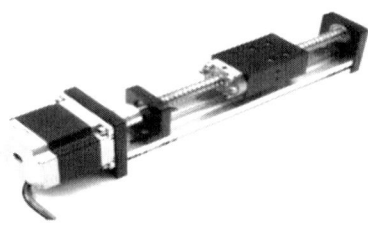

Figure 17. Threaded rod linear guide rail.

- Linear Potentiometer: It used for linear position or displacement measurements. In this prototype, it is placed inside the syringe's holder to measure the size of the syringe being placed as shown in Figure 18.

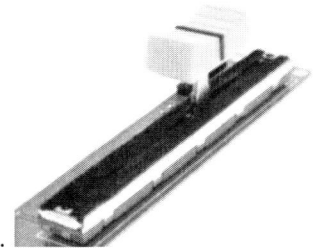

Figure 18. Linear potentiometer.

- Rotary Encoder: A rotary encoder, shown in Figure 19, is both an electrical and mechanical device that changes the angular position or motion of a shaft to an analog or digital signal.

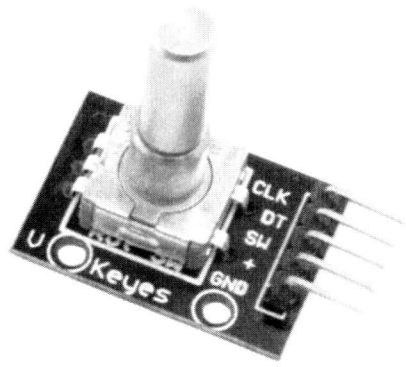

Figure 19. Rotary encoder.

- Limit Switch: It is an electro-mechanical device, shown in Figure 20, used to continue or break an electrical connection. It consists of an actuator that is mechanically connected to a set of contacts. It is used in this system for calibration and detection of the drug volume inside the syringe.

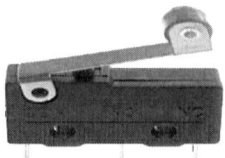

Figure 20. Limit switch.

- Nextion LCD 7 inch LCD: It is a Human Machine Interface (HMI) solution that provides control and visualization interface between an individual and a process, machine, application or appliance. It is used to display the patient's information and collected results. Figure 21 shows this type of LCD.

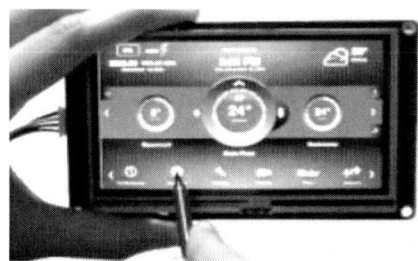

Figure 21. Nextion 7" LCD.

The prototype connections of all these components cited previously are shown in Figure 22 using a simple breadboard.

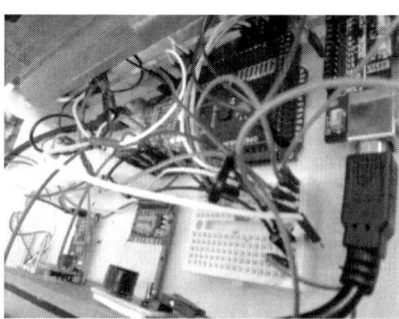

Figure 22. Prototype testing on breadboard.

METHODOLOGY AND IMPLEMENTATION

The only requirement for the smart self-monitored syringe infusion pump is the calibration (placement and/or removal) of the syringe by the nurse. All data will be sent to a central station to be monitored by the staff, and consequently to EMR (Electronic Medical Record) system. An alarm system is also added in case of any error or misreading caused by the sensors connected to the patient monitor. This functioning process is shown in Figure 23.

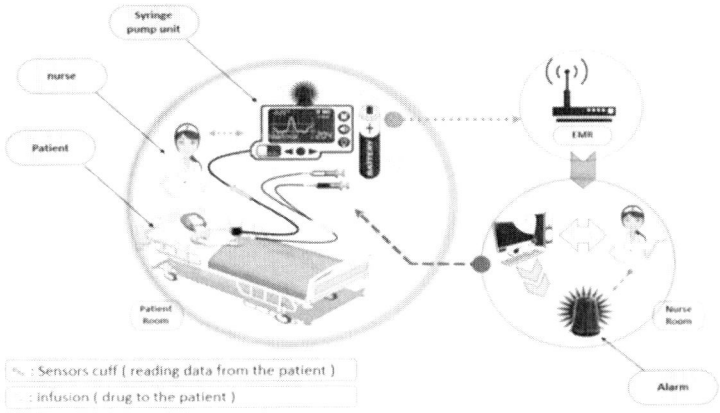

Figure 23. An illustrative image showing how the prototype works.

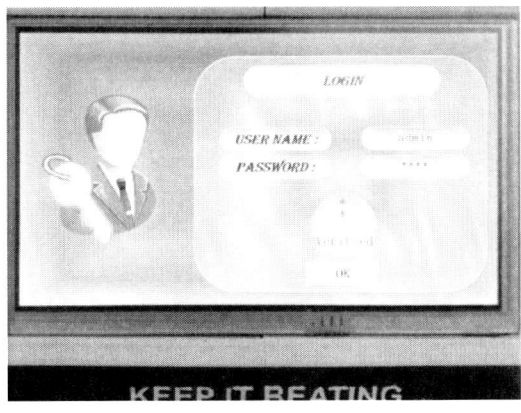

Figure 24. Logging in to the system.

As mentioned before, the main objective behind this system is to reduce the nurses' workload and also to reduce the errors caused by medical staff. Therefore, the only thing should be done by the nurse is to place the syringe having the appropriate drug inside the syringe holder and to fill all the needed information related to the patient (name, age, drug name, date, etc.) on the display screen using his/her credentials as shown in Figures 24 and 25.

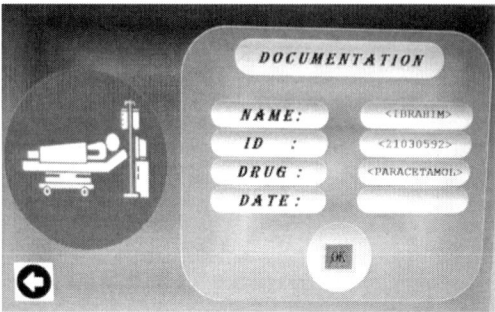

Figure 25. Entering Patient's Information.

The syringe holder contains a linear potentiometer inside, connected to the controller (Arduino) to detect the size of the placed syringe. This holder is compatible with all syringe sizes. Also, the arm which is adhered to the movable part of the linear guide rail that moves the plunger of the syringe contains a limit switch. The zero references are set constant for all syringe sizes at the end of the guide rail. When the arm moves from the reference, the limit switch will be pressed when the arm reaches the plunger.

The encoder connected to the linear guide rail measures the distance (d) passed from zero reference until the limit switch inside the arm. The volume of the syringe will be calculated according to the equation of the cylinder's volume:

$$V = \pi r^2 L \tag{1}$$

where L is the maximum length of the selected syringe subtracted from the measured distance (d).

A drug library that contains information about most common drugs given by syringe pump is added to limit the flow range of the administrated drug.

All sensors, that replaced the patient monitor, are connected to two Arduino controllers. The first one (NANO) is used as a master and the second one (MEGA) as a slave. Reading data is acquired using an Arduino code with multi libraries and reading specific functions in order to control the flow of drug according to the acquired readings. All these connections are shown in the block diagram of Figure 26.

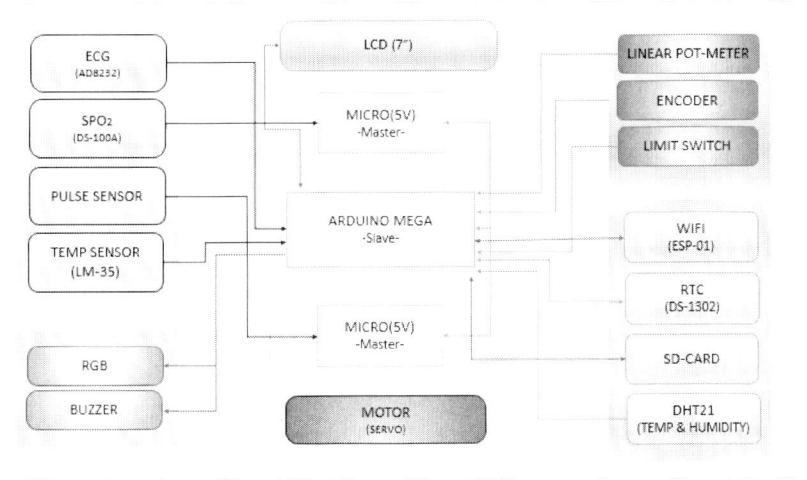

Figure 26. Block diagram showing the components' connections.

Safety

The safety is most important issue to think about as well known any medical device must be safe for everyone.

Also, electrical safety should be well considered to eliminate any harm that could threaten the patient's life. This device is considered as a class II since the power is driven from 5V USB cable according to the International Electro-technical Commission (IEC) standard and guidelines.

Implementation Tools

Several tools were used to accomplish this prototype, especially for the hardware design:

- 3D Printer: Cetus 3D printer was used to print out all plastic cases of the system using different colors of plastic filaments.
- Fusion 360: It is an Autodesk program used to draw the 3D parts of the design in order to be inserted in the cetus3D program to the printout.
- 3D Builder: IT is also used to draw 3D components and make sure of the measurements and scales in mm.
- Nextion Editor: It is used for programming of the Nextion screen with the ability to add different icons' shapes.
- ECG Pads: They are electrodes placed on the skin after adding a gel to record the electrical activity of the heart as PQRST signal.

Implementation Summary

Each component was programmed alone with a specific code using Arduino language. The programmed Nextion LCD was very useful to enter the patient needed information and his/her situation and to hold inside a drug library with most important drugs given invasively. It is always updated and displayed the output results and signals. The overall prototype is shown in Figure 27.

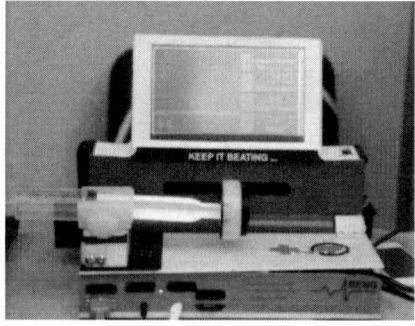

Figure 27. The final design.

Test Cases and Acceptance Criteria

After logging into the system using the nurse user credential (Username and Password), the nurse has to fill the patient's information (name, age, gender, height, etc.) as shown in Figure 28.

Figure 29 shows the patient's room temperature and humidity including parameters and signals taken from temperature and humidity sensors.

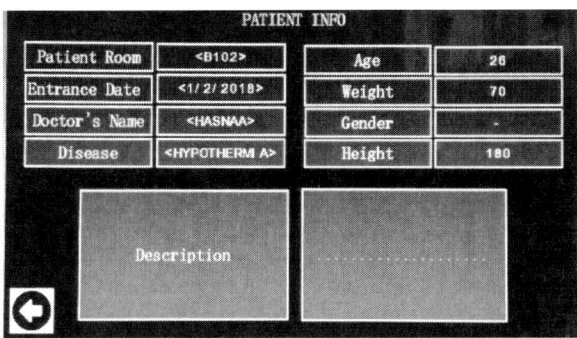

Figure 28. Patient's information.

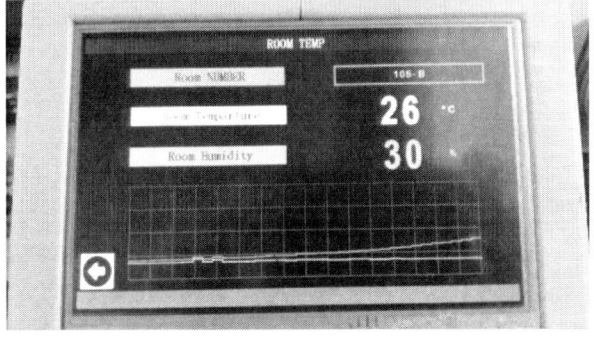

Figure 29. Room temperature & humidity range.

A member of our team was chosen as a candidate to test ECG, SpO2, heart beat rate and temperature. Three ECG electrodes were placed on his chest to record his heart's activity. SpO2 and temperature sensors were placed on his finger. The output signals and readings the acquired data are shown in Figure 30 in addition to the drug's flow, volume and time. Note that the flow is calculated based on the following equation:

$$Flow = \frac{Volume}{Time} \qquad (2)$$

The ECG signals were better collected and displayed when downloading to the system (microcontroler) an optimized and dedicated program as shown in Figure 31.

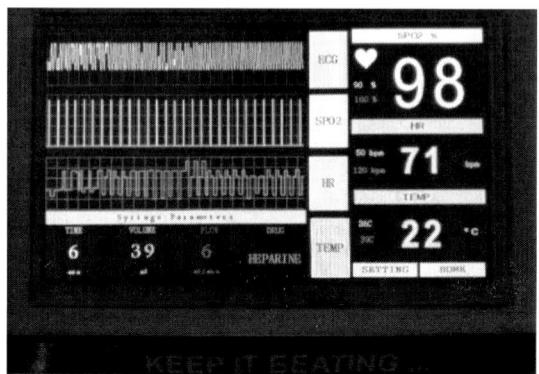

Figure 30. Graphical and numerical values in patient monitor's screen.

Figure 31. Graphical ECG Signal.

When Paracetamol drug was selected by the user, the system will directly display its limits on the LCD with information regarding this drug obtained from the library, as shown in Figure 32. In addition, some parameters were calculated and displayed on the screen such as the maximum and minimum limits of the flow rate and the infusion time, and maximum limit of volume. When zeros are displayed for the volume, flow, time and syringe size, this indicates that the syringe arm is in calibration process. This means that the system did not reach the syringe plunger to detect its size and to start the administration.

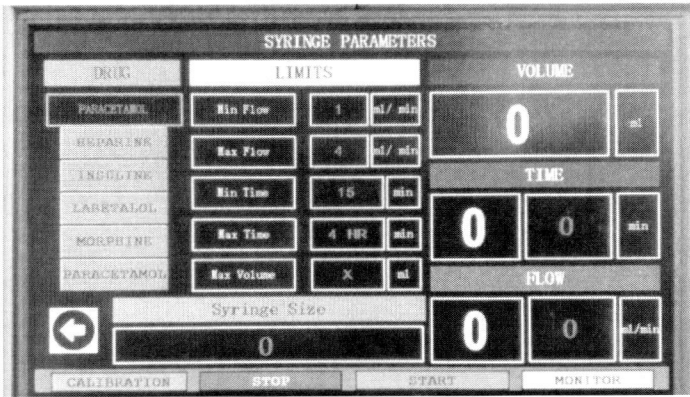

Figure 32. Pre-calibration syringe pump's screenshot.

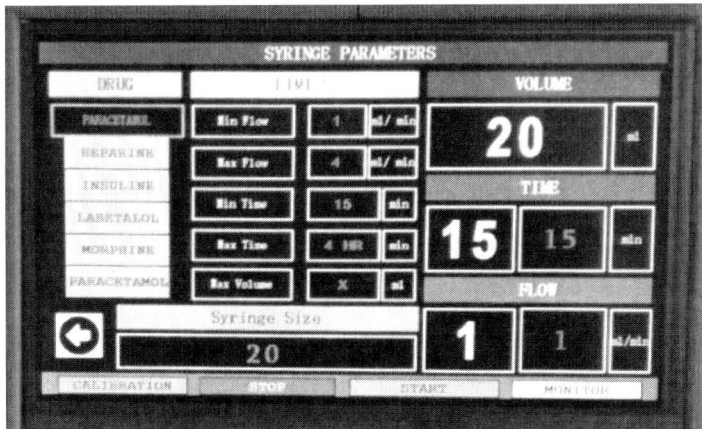

Figure 33. Post-calibration syringe pump's screenshot.

While in Figure 33, the calibration was done and the start button is pressed. The syringe size was detected as 20 ml in addition to the calculated flow from volume and time.

CONCLUSION AND FUTURE WORKS

The patient's safety becomes a major concern and a top priority in the design and manufacturing of medical equipments in addition to other challenges in such field. The prototype proposed in this paper comes as a part of an effort to provide and support such safe practice as well as to treat the problem of the shortage in the medical staff, and the high cost created as a practical outcome of such problem. Moreover, a possible outcome of this proposed smart syringe infusion pump integrated system is to reduce the morbidity and mortality rate as well as the support of more intelligent automation and integration in the intensive care environments for the benefits of both the patients and the healthcare contributors.

Every important and beneficial system should undergo continuous improvement to track and go after new technologies and inventions to stay up to date especially if it is related to medical equipments that can contribute to enhancing people's life.

The smart self-monitored syringe infusion pump can be modified and improved by taking the followings into considertation:

- Invasive blood pressure port can be added to measure blood pressure invasively which is considered more accurate.
- The programming code can be enhanced by adding specific functions to allow the system to auto-calibrate itself permanently to determine, check and rectify its measurements' graduation according to specific references. The calibration of the threaded rod linear guide rail has been already achieved by adding the null start of all syringe sizes.
- Continuous update of drug library by adding new drugs and maximizing the memory storage to accommodate a large number of drugs.
- The idea of this system can be applied to multi syringe and infusion pumps i.e., pumps station.

- The communication can be applied to all machines placed in ICU leading to a fully smart area.

REFERENCES

[1] Marshall, J. (2017). "What is an intensive care unit? A report of the task force of the World Federation of Societies of Intensive and Critical Care Medicine," *Journal of Critical Care*, vol. 37, p. 270–276,.

[2] Hettinger, B. J. and Brazile, R. P. (2019). "Health Level Seven (HL7): standard for healthcare electronic data transmissions.," *Current neurology and neuroscience reports.*, 1994. [Online]. Available: https://www.ncbi.nlm.nih.gov/pubmed/8149297. [Accessed: 04-Feb-2019].

[3] Wiklund, M. E. (2019). "Making Medical Device Interfaces More User-Friendly," MDDI Online, 07-Aug-2017. [Online]. Available: https://www.mddionline.com/making-medical-device-interfaces-more-user-friendly. [Accessed: 04-Feb-2019].

[4] Alaris™ CC Plus Syringe Pump with Guardrails™ Safety Software," Becton Dickinson. [online] Available at: https://www.bd.com/en-uk/products/infusion/infusion-devices/alaris-plus-platform-with-guardrails-safety-software/alaris-cc-plus-syringe-pump-with-guardrails [Accessed: 4 Feb. 2019].

[5] "IntelliVue MX550 Portable/bedside patient monitor," Philips. [Online]. Available: https://www.usa.philips.com/healthcare/product/HC866066/intellivue-mx550-patient-monitor. [Accessed: 04-Feb-2019].

[6] Sprunk, N., Garcia, A. M., Schreiber, U., Bauernschmitt, R. and Knoll, A. (2011). "Cardiovascular model for development and test of automated hemodynamic regulation with medication," *Computing in Cardiology*, p. 153–156.

[7] Sprunk, N. *et al.* (2011). "Hemodynamic regulation using fuzzy logic," *2011 Eighth International Conference on Fuzzy Systems and Knowledge Discovery (FSKD)*, p. 515-519.

[8] Mendoza, G. A. *et al.* (2011). "Automation of an extracorporeal support system with adaptive fuzzy controllers," *2011 Annual International Conference of the IEEE Engineering in Medicine and Biology Society*, p. 1033-1036.

[9] Haddad, W. M., Bailey, J. M., Hayakawa, T. and Hovakimyan, N. (2007). "Neural Network Adaptive Output Feedback Control for Intensive Care Unit Sedation and Intraoperative Anesthesia," in *IEEE Transactions on Neural Networks*, vol. 18, no. 4, p. 1049-1066.

[10] Padhye, N. S., Hamlin, S., Brazdeikis, A. and S. Hanneman, K. (2009). "Cardiovascular impact of manual and automated turns in ICU," *2009 Annual International Conference of the IEEE Engineering in Medicine and Biology Society*, Minneapolis, MN, p. 1844-1847.

[11] Sprunk, N., Kaur, M., Bauernschmitt, R., Mendoza G. A. and Knoll, A. (2012). "System design for simultaneous data acquisition from patient monitor and syringe pumps in intensive care unit," *2012 IEEE-EMBS Conference on Biomedical Engineering and Sciences*, Langkawi, p. 878-882.

In: Vital Signs: An Overview
Editors: Roy Abi Zeid Daou et al.
ISBN: 978-1-53617-765-7
© 2020 Nova Science Publishers, Inc.

Chapter 5

IMPLEMENTATION OF A MONITORING SYSTEM THAT NOTIFIES HEALTHCARE PROVIDERS OF A SUDDEN MEDICAL EMERGENCY OCCURRING TO A DRIVER

Joseph Khattar[1], Carla Zeine[1], Roy Abi Zeid Daou[1,2],*, Ali Hayek[3] and Josef Boercsoek[3]

[1]Lebanese German University, Public Health Faculty,
Biomedical Technologies Department, Jounieh, Lebanon
[2]Mart, Learning, Education and Research Center, Chananiir, Lebanon
[3]Kassel University,
Institute of Computer Architecture and System Programming,
Kassel, Germany

ABSTRACT

In many car accident cases, the problem is pretty straightforward: the other driver ran a red light, or couldn't stop in time and rear-ended the

---

* Corresponding Author's Email: r.abizeiddaou@lgu.edu.lb.

other vehicle, for example. However, in situations where the other driver suffered a medical emergency just before the accident, liability is not so simple.

In this chapter, the main objective is to limit car accidents caused due to a medical emergency. This would require the use of some vital sign sensors to continuously measure the medical parameters of the drivers and notify the health care providers as well as the nearby cars of any medical problem facing the driver.

The main target is to implement some sensors that measure the main vital signs of a driver, in a non-invasive and comfortable way in order not to affect his activity. Thus, as an alternative solution for the wearable equipment, some sensors have been integrated within the driving wheel. Furthermore, Arduinos were used as the main processing units and the MAX3010x SPO2/HR dual sensors have been implemented in order to measure the driver's heart rate and the SPO2 (Blood Oxygen Saturation Rate) values. Some alarms have been added physically and others were integrated in a phone application. This latter has two profiles: the health care provider profile that gets notified whenever the measured parameters are indeed outside the already set thresholds and the user profile which is used to enable alarms and/or notify the driver of any problem or misuse of the system.

The system was tested by more than 10 persons (for more than two hours for each test) having different health problems and the system delivered no false alarms. As for the accuracy of the system, each sensor output has been compared to an already existent system as the case of the NIBP for example and all tests have been achieved successfully. Added to that, the system was tested on several car manufacturers, models and brands.

Keywords: car drivers, vital signs measurement, heart rate, SPO2, phone application, safe system, location detection, cardiovascular diseases, diabetes disease

1. INTRODUCTION

The main reasons that have led to the realization of this system are to solve the problem of car accidents due to emergency medical problems. In fact, the below questions are rising in today's world: *Can the medical emergency events during driving be detected to prevent greater damage?*

What are the actions that could be done in order to limit the effects of cardiac or diabetic dysfunction among drivers on road accidents? What is the effect of adding a smart vital signs monitoring system to vehicles on reducing road accidents associated with driver's medical problems?

These questions are of a great importance. Similar questions were asked in a report achieved by the *National Highway Traffic Safety Administration* in 2009 [1]. Moreover, while on the road, people may experience different medical issues, especially if they are already diagnosed with a certain disease such as diabetes or heart diseases. Studies show that driving on the road may be very dangerous for these types of people and for the other cars around them as shown in Table 1. It has been noted that, between 2005 and 2007 in the U.S., 20% of medical conditions reported in crashes were due to diabetic reactions, 35% percent were caused by seizures and 11% were caused by heart attacks [2] [3].

Thus, the main idea of the project is to develop a monitoring and alarm system able to detect abnormalities in some vital signs in such an easy way that does not confuse the driver while driving and force him indirectly to be using it for safety considerations. In other words, the implemented system will not cause any harm or frustration for the driver while letting him measure his vital signs easily. The features of the proposed system allow informing concerned persons of the driver actual status and the car location in case of medical status abnormality.

Table 1. Types of medical conditions responsible for crashes [2]

Medical Condition	Estimated Count	Unweighted Count	Estimated Percent
Seizure	17,222	48	35%
Black Out	14,217	37	29%
Diabetic Reaction	9,963	30	20%
Heart Attack	5,288	9	11%
Stroke	1,261	7	3%
Other	1,918	7	4%
Total	49,868	138	100%

Source: NMVCCS July 2005 to December 2007

In more details, the main objective of the proposed system is to monitor and analyze the vital signs of the driver while driving in order to limit or reduce road accidents resulting from medical issues and to save lives of other drivers. Moreover, this system should provide an indirect minor health checkup that helps in detecting early signs of underlying health problems.

Once an abnormal status is recorded, an SMS and a notification will be sent to the health care professionals along with the actual position of the person (or the car) in order to act as soon as possible and to reduce the mortality probability. A button can be pressed by the driver in order to remove/suspend the alarm. Another alarm will be turned on to inform nearby cars of the problem facing the driver of the concerned car.

This chapter will be divided as follow: section 2 will present the block diagram of the system whereas section will show the most relevant papers discussing this problem. In section 4, the hardware tools used will be presented whereas is section 5, the software running the processing units and the phone application will be shown. Section 6 will present the implementation and the validation processes. At the end, section 7 will conclude this work and proposes some ideas to enhance the system.

2. BLOCK DIAGRAM

The block diagram of the system shows the functionalities along with the technical choices taken during the design and implementation phases. Thus, Figure 1 shows the block diagram of the system along with the hardware components. The processing unit is the brain of this system. All sensors and alarms are connected to this electrical chip.

On the other side, the sensors are placed on the driving wheel in order to offer the maximum comfort to the driver. Two sensors are used in order to increase the safety architecture of the system and to limit the false alarms. The driver has only to put his finger on the sensor for about 8 seconds in order to get the HR and the SPO2 values. In fact, this time is a bit long but during this frame, the sensor is reading multiple values and is calculating the average value for better accuracy.

As for the alarms, when an abnormal measurement is encountered and is maintained for a certain time, several alarms are generated. The first one is within the car to inform the driver that he has a health issue. The latter can press a button (for a certain time) to remove the alarm. In case no actions were taken, the location of the car will be sent to the healthcare provider along with some information about the driver (his profile and his current health status) in order to act as soon as possible. The data analysis and display is done through a phone application consisting of two interfaces: the driver profile and the healthcare professional profile.

However, to achieve a certain safety integrity level according to international safety standards, especially for safety standards applied in the medical and automotive field, several safety-related measures need to be implemented along all the development life cycle of the presented concept. Therefore, several requirements of the relevant standards should be met at sensor level, microcontroller level as well as at actor or output level. Since this work presents a first concept of the target application, safety measures are not applied at this stage of the implementation. For future work a risk analysis and a detailed safety concept according to the relevant standards will be developed and analyzed. In this context, the main measures will focus on applying redundancy, diversity as well as testability issues and monitoring units to all the components of the presented system, in order to enhance the reliability, the availability and the safety of the target application. Furthermore several evaluation and estimation work will be carried out to assess the safety-related parameters. The safety concept and its evaluation process will be published in a future research work.

3. STATE OF THE ART

Prior surveys and systems on the topics of medical emergencies detection while driving have been published. However, the field is considered as a brand new hot topic, since it hasn't been explored yet.

Several researchers have reviewed and design systems for an embedded system but failed to develop one or faced major complications. The two giant automotive companies, FORD and BMW, just started working on such projects recently and are still in the first stages of their projects [4] [5].

This section will be divided into two parts: in the first one, the vital signs measurements and thresholds will be presented whereas in the second part, the monitoring systems embedded within the car will be shown.

3.1. Vital Signs Systems

Talib et al. proposed a system to help elderly people in the UAE. The system comprises a device that includes sensors as the Heart Rate (HR) measurement module, a smartphone based mobile unit for review with doctor, and a healthcare database server for data recording and backup. An Arduino microcontroller was used to analyze signals. Normal and abnormal ranges for vital signs were set. When signals are outside the normal range, an alarm will sound to alert the healthcare providers and a SMS will be sent to a specific person to ask for help. A short report of the abnormality will be sent to the cloud for processing and forwarded to the nearest hospital to ask for assistance. The sensors are placed in a wearable object such as shirts or watches. The results show the outcome of each sensor alone but didn't mention the accuracy, the reliability and the response time of this system [6].

Constant et al. proposed a system that is able to measure the HR by wearing special glasses, called pulse glasses. The system could be also connected to the cloud and it serves as a part of the Internet of Things (IoT). As for the results, it was tested over one person only and it was compared to the output of the Electrocardiogram (ECG). The authors showed that the system still needs to do additional hardware implementation, mainly filtering [7].

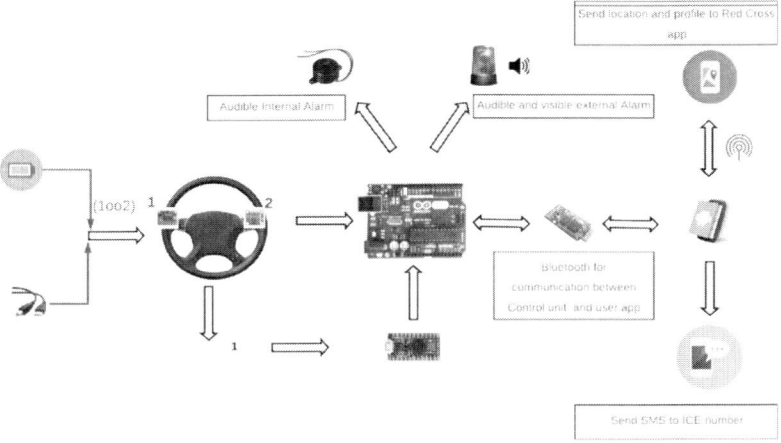

Figure 1. Block diagram of the proposed system.

Another recent study, conducted by Chandrasekhar et al., proposed a novel method to measure the Blood Pressure (BP) by using the oscillometric finger-pressing method of the smart phone. Thus, inflatable cuffs were not used; they were replaced by the measurement of the finger pressure on the smartphone. During these instances, the phone would measure the applied pressure and the resulting variable amplitude blood volume oscillations. The system was tested by 30 persons and was compared to the standard cuff-based device. Bias and precision errors were recorded; however, the authors concluded that such system may be feasible using smartphones [8].

Added to these researchers, several scientific papers have been published related to the measurement of vital signs in order to continuously check the health of any person. Interested readers can check the following references [9] [10] [11].

3.2. Cars Embedded Systems

The system proposed by Jung et al. is an ECG based driver's health monitoring system. The sensors are composed from an active electrode, a ground electrode and a wireless sensor node. The electrodes are placed as follow: the active electrode is placed on the front of the car seat where the driver lays his back. The ground electrode is placed on the car seat where he sits and finally, the wireless node is placed on the back of the car seat. Once the system is set, it can start monitoring the ECG of the driver and then transmit the signals to the server through the wireless node for analysis. After analysis, the server determines the current health state, if it's normal, experiencing fatigue or drowsiness [12].

Singh et al. suggested a non-contact method to monitor heartbeat signals with ECG. This method consists of implementing several ECG electrodes on the car seat of the driver in order to monitor continuously the changes, independently of the driver's sitting position, his mass or any other variables. The readings of the signals are done by using digital signal processing methods that help with rendering reliable real-time health monitoring [13].

Lee et al. proposed a health monitor system implemented in cars based on non-contact and non-pressurized sensors in order to offer to the driver the maximum comfort. The system has been implemented within the seat belt facing the chest/heart of the driver and the measured results have visualized his heart rate. Almost the same results were obtained while using the ECG device with an error of about 3% [14].

4. HARDWARE COMPONENTS

In this section, the different physical tools used to realize and implement the proposed system will be proposed. Hence, the sensors, the processing units, the communication tools and the power supply module will be presented.

4.1. Sensors

Medically, the most important vital signs are the electrical activity of the heart (ECG), the Blood Pressure (BP), the Blood Oxygen Saturation

(SPO2), the Respiratory Rate (RR) and the Heart Rate (HR) [15]. Monitoring these parameters requires the presence of sensors capable of measuring them in a non-invasive and comfortable way.

Since the car environment will handle this device, the various noise sources present will strongly affect the sensitive measurements as the ECG and the BP. On the other hand, despite the high cost of the high sensitivity ECG electrodes, the comfort of the driver using this system highly matters. So, the ECG, the BP and the RR were excluded since their measurements require the presence of external wearable stuff as well as a perfect isolated environment that is not so efficient in cars due to the humps, the bumps and the other road obstacles.

Also, as we are dealing with a medical system, the precision, the response time (in milliseconds) and the error rate of the sensors are values of great importance and must be considered when choosing the sensors.

Taking all these requirements in account, and aiming to use low cost, small size, noise sensitive features as well as safe and reliable considerations, the two series of the **High-Sensitivity Pulse Oximeter and Heart-Rate Sensor (Max30100 and MAX30105)** were chosen to measure the HR and the SPO2 of the driver.

The MAX30100 sensor (shown in Figure 2.a) consists of two LEDs, one emitting a red light, another emitting infrared (IR) light. For pulse rate, only the infrared light is needed. Both the red light and infrared light are used to measure oxygen levels in blood. When the heart pumps blood, there is an increase in oxygenated blood as a result of having more blood. As the heart relaxes, the volume of oxygenated blood also decreases. When identifying the time between the increase and decrease of oxygenated blood, the pulse rate is determined [16]. This sensor operates on 1.8V power supply so it will not work with microcontrollers with higher logic levels such as the Arduino as its delivered voltage ranges between 3.3V and 5V. Thus, some modifications on its board were done to make it operates on 5V.

As for the MAX30105 sensor (represented in Figure 2.b), it has the same electrical constitution of the MAX30100; however, it has also a smoke detection feature and it make several internal measurements before delivering the SPO2 and the HR values.

The main features of both sensors are the followings:

- Complete Pulse Oximeter and Heart-Rate Sensor Solution Simplifies Design:
  - Integrated LEDs, Photo Sensor, and High-Performance Analog Front - End;
  - Tiny 5.6mm x 2.8mm x 1.2mm 14-Pin Optically Enhanced System-in-Package;
- Ultra-Low-Power Operation Increases Battery Life for Wearable Devices:
  - Programmable Sample Rate and LED Current for Power Savings;
  - Ultra-Low Shutdown Current (0.7µA);
- Advanced Functionality Improves Measurement Performance:
  - High SNR Provides Robust Motion Artifact Resilience;
  - Integrated Ambient Light Cancellation;
  - High Sample Rate Capability;
  - Fast Data Output Capability;

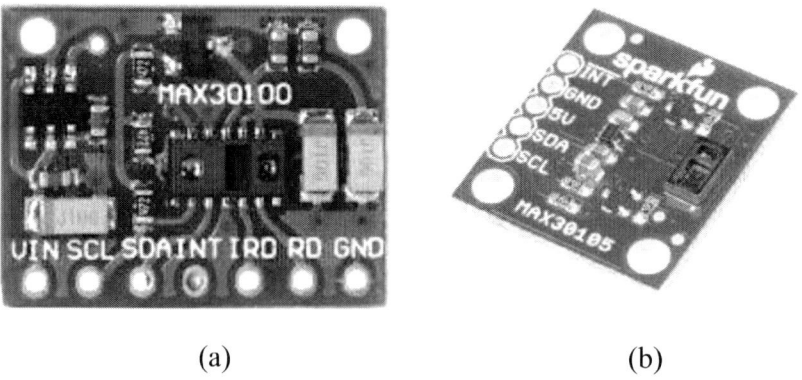

(a) (b)

Figure 2. Images of the MAX30100 (a) and MAX30105 (b) sensors.

4.2. Communication Interface

The communication is a main part of this system. It is needed in order to send alarms to health care professionals. Several communication protocols could be used as WiFi, GSM and Bluetooth. The main objective of this module is to enable sending alarms and data from the processing unit in case of emergency problem as well as sharing the location of the car.

The HC-06 module (shown in Figure 3) is an easy to use Bluetooth Serial Port Protocol (SSP) module, designed for transparent wireless serial connection setup. This module is fully qualified Bluetooth V2.0+ Enhanced Data Rate (EDR), 3Mbps Modulation with complete 2.4GHz radio transceiver and baseband. It uses CSR Blue core 04-External single chip Bluetooth system with CMOS technology and with AFH (Adaptive Frequency Hopping) feature [17].

The main features of this communication system are the following:

- Typical -80dBm sensitivity;
- Up to +4dBm RF transmit power;
- Low Power 1.8V Operation, 1.8 to 3.6V I/O;
- PIO control;
- UART interface with programmable baud rate;
- Equipped with an integrated antenna of 2.4GHz;

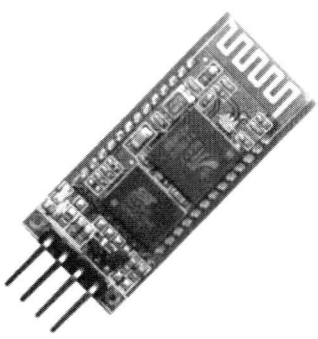

Figure 3. HC06 Bluetooth module electronic board.

4.3. Processing Unit

Many types of processing units can be found on the market and they have different purposes and different ways of programing. From among these devices, one can list the PIC Microcontroller developed by Microchip, the Raspberry PI kit that encloses several functionalities and features controlled by a processor, the Arduino microcontrollers, the PLC, the Data Acquisition board (DAQ) of National Instruments along with LabView software which enables the inputs and outputs to/from the software to monitor and control the electrical circuit, and much more.

For this system, as one of the important requirements is its low cost and small size, the Arduino microcontroller has been chosen. In fact, two Arduino microcontrollers will be used, each one connected to a MAX sensor. This design was chosen in order to increase the safety of the system by implementing redundant sub-systems and to limit the false alarms. In fact, each processing unit calculates the vital signs apart. Whenever the values measured in both sensors are outside the normal ranges, an alarm will be generated. Along with the above mentioned safety concept, microcontroller units which are designed and certified for use in medical and automotive applications could be part of a future work to improve the safety of the overall system.

The operational code implemented of these processing units will be presented in details in the next section.

4.4. Power Supply Module

The last puzzle piece of the hardware components is the power supply module. Two power supply sources were implemented. The primary option was to connect the system to the car power supply input and to use a 5V regulator (the 7805 IC) in order to limit the supply voltage of the processing unit and the sensors. The second option consists of using a 9V battery that serves as a backup in case the car's battery level becomes low.

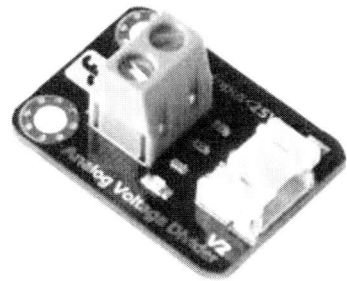

Figure 4. Voltage divider board to monitor the battery level.

In fact, as the system power consumption does not exceed few milli-ampers, the choice of a power supply unit was not very complicated as any option would last for a long time.

However, to remain fully functional, an option was added on the phone application module to display the battery level (when using the second option) and to notify the user whenever this supply unit needs to be replaced. The circuitry used to achieve this testing consists of the use of a voltage divider module as shown in Figure 4.

5. SOFTWARE TOOLS

After showing all the hardware components needed for the design of the monitoring system, this section will describe the software tools and flowcharts applied for the good functioning of the system. Hence, this section will be divided into two parts: in the first one, the code running the processing units will be provided whereas, in the second part, the phone application responsible to communicate with the health care provider and to deliver notifications will be presented.

5.1. Microcontrollers Code

As already presented in the hardware section, two Arduino microcontrollers were used where each one was connected to a MAX sensor. Thus, the basic functionality of both microcontrollers is the same: continuously reading the sensor's values for a defined time interval, compute the average values, compare these values to certain thresholds and generate alarms when needed.

The flowchart of Figure 5 illustrates the general working principle of the whole system. The implemented method consists of reading the HR value coming from the first sensor using the first microcontroller whereas the second microcontroller reads the HR and the SPO2 values coming from the second sensor. The main issue that limited the reading of the SPO2 form the MAX30105 sensor is the memory space capacity required for this value processing which exceed the storage size of the Arduino. Both values are then compared using any microcontroller after sharing these values between the two microcontrollers. The decision will be shown in the flowcharts of Figures 6 and 7.

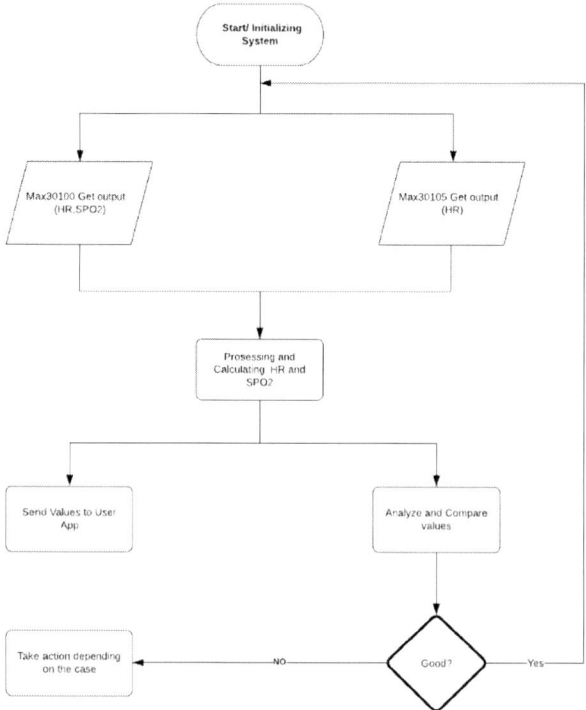

Figure 5. General flowchart of the Arduino program.

Here, two cases are mainly to be considered when using both sensors:

1. One or both Heart Rate Measurements are Zeros

In the first case (Figure 6), if one or both HR values are equal to zero for a period of time – set by the user – then, most probably, the user is not using the sensor (his fingers are not connected to the MAX3010x). Either he/she is holding the driving wheel in a wrong way or facing a bad situation and is not able to handle it. Moreover, a possible problem could reside in the hardware itself: the user may be placing hands correctly but the system/sensor is down.

Through the phone application, the user selects what is called the Refresh Time (RF). The RF is the time differences between the first zero measurement and the last one before alarming the user to place both fingers for a checkup.

After the RF passes, an oral notification from the application will alert the user to place fingers on the sensors. If the user does not respond, the alarm will continue to appear for one minute. In case of continuous negative feedback, the app will ask the user if he/she is OK. The NO answer (the *NO* button of the phone application is pressed) or the absence of answer for a specific time will mean that the driver needs help.

Therefore, the app will send the driver's location and profile to the health care provider and a SMS to the ICE specified number at the same time. An external audible alarm with LEDs will also notify the surrounding cars to be aware. On the other hand, pressing YES will return the system to its normal functioning state and the parameters will be recalculated normally.

Moreover, if this condition is repeated for four consecutive times and the answer is YES every time, then the user is in good health and the system may be down and in need for maintenance. Therefore, another oral notification will inform the user about the system status and the Bluetooth connection with the system will be disconnected.

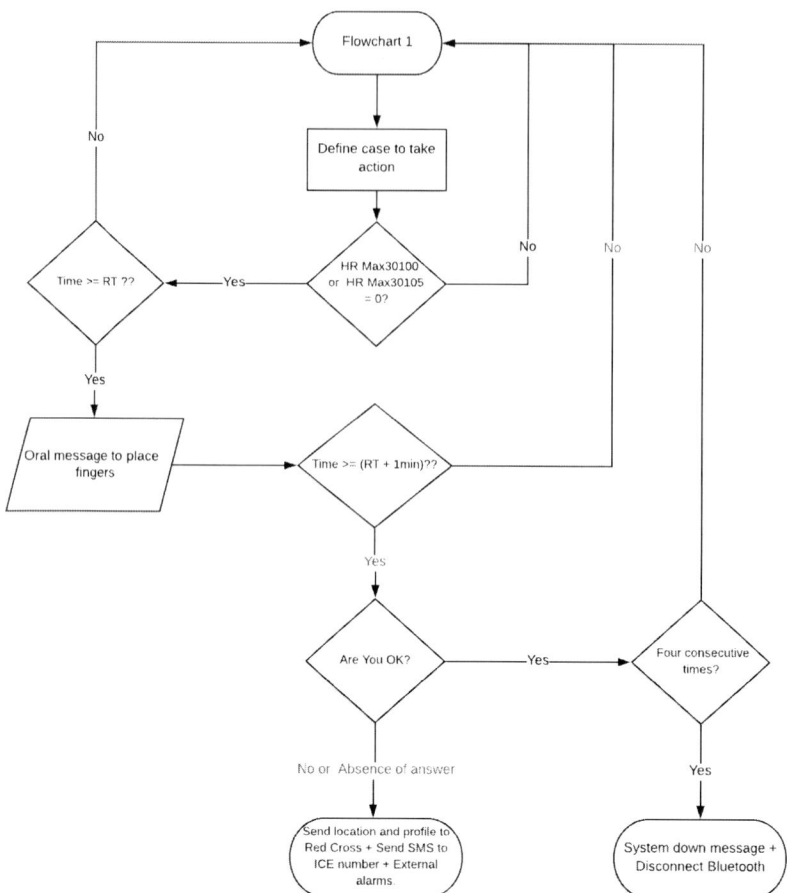

Figure 6. Flowchart of the first case.

2. *One or both HR Measurements are Out of the Defined Thresholds*

For the second case, when the heart rate value exceeds the upper or lower acceptable rate[1], and since it is a dual check redundant system, the system will check the SPO2 value. If this latter is abnormal along with the HR for about 16 seconds, the driver then is most probably suffering a serious issue. The "ARE YOU OK?" message will alert the user and the same procedure as in the previous case will follow it.

---

[1] No references indicate the upper and lower heart rate values. However, based on some medical doctors experience, we have fixed the lower rate to 40 beats per minute (BPM) and the higher one to 140 BPM

On the other hand, if the SPO2 is within the normal range, the app will notify the user to adjust his fingers placement as the abnormal values of the HR may be due to the presence of many unpredictable noise sources in the car environment or due to a fault in such a low cost sensor. Added to that, if this alarm is repeated for six times, the system will disconnect the Bluetooth connection and the need for maintenance will be announced. Figure 7 shows the flowchart of this case.

5.2. Phone Application

The MIT App Inventor, which is an intuitive, visual programming environment that allows nonprofessionals to build fully functional apps for smartphones and tablets, was used. Its blocks-based tool facilitates the creation of complex, high-impact apps in significantly less time than traditional programming environments [18].

The mobile application is set up for two interfaces: the healthcare provider and the driver. The mobile application is used for display and also control of some major features. Since we have two categories of users using the application and need to communicate together, a connection was created to allow query-retrieve between the two different pages using APIs (Application Programming Interface). Figure 8 shows some print screens of the phone application.

6. IMPLEMENTATION AND VALIDATION

In this part, the electric circuit grouping the sensors, the microcontrollers, the connection and the power supplies will be shown together. Thus, Figure 9 shows the whole electrical part of this system drawn using Fritzing and implemented on a breadboard.

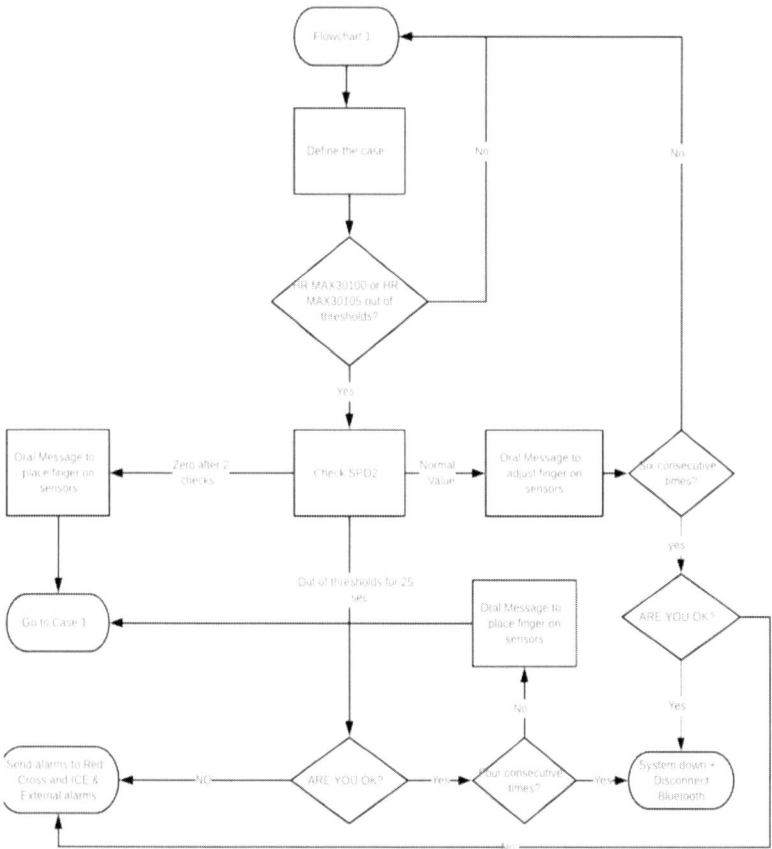

Figure 7. Flowchart of the second case.

The MAX3010X sensors require I²C communication ports. As each Arduino Uno has one SDA (Serial Data) and one SCL (Serial clock line), each sensor is connected to a microcontroller. These two Arduinos communicate together using the software serial communication to free the Tx/Rx pins; these latter being used for the Bluetooth module.

The software serial communication was used in order to solve a major problem: the connection between the two Arduinos each having its own functional sensor (the MAX3010x) can be done using the Rx/Tx pins. However, the need of the Bluetooth module has led to free these pins and the use of the software serial communication.

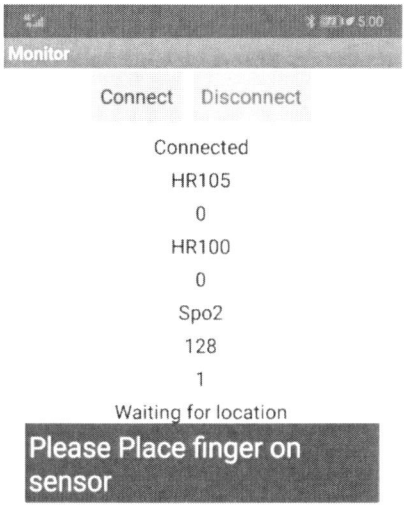
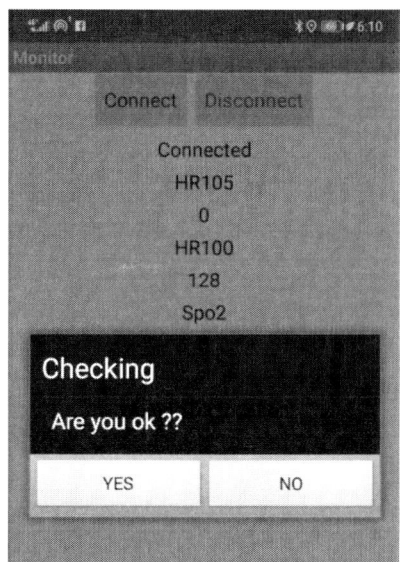

Figure 8. Print screen of the phone application.

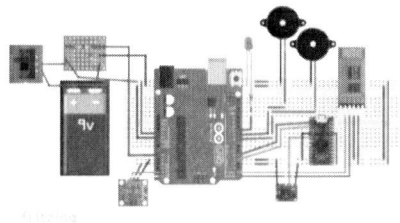
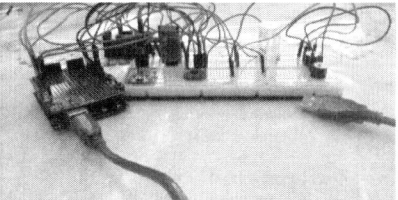

Figure 9. Circuit assembly design and implementation.

As for the communication module with the phone application, the Bluetooth HC-06 device was used. This communication tool is responsible for the serial communication via the Tx and Rx pins of the Arduino with the mobile application.

Two audible alarms were deployed: one for internal use to notify the driver to place his fingers on the sensors and the other, coupled with LEDs, to serve for the external alarm to warn other drivers when a medical problem is recorded.

Added to that, the filtering of the signal acquired by the MAX sensors was realized using two approaches: a hardware pre-filtering and amplification technique that removes the noise caused by the car vibration and software filtering to limit the interference of the infrared generated by the sensor with the light for better accuracy.

As for the power, a 9V battery was used although the system can be connected to the Radio USB of the car. A small electronic circuit is added to calculate the capacity of the battery and to check its lifecycle. This value is also sent to the application and displayed on main screen.

At the end, the sensors are mounted on the steering wheel of a car in the 3 o'clock and 9 o'clock positions [19] [20]. Figures 10 show the exact position of the sensors.

As for the validation, a much reduced number of errors occurred at the level of the measurements. These errors were mainly due to the low cost of the sensors. In order to reduce the effects of these errors, some codes were added as reading several consecutive values of the sensors and calculating the average before comparing them to the thresholds.

Thus, to make sure of the good functioning of the sensors, their values were compared to Non-Invasive Blood Pressure (NIBP) machine. Figure 11 compares both outputs. It is clear that due to the applied filters and codes, both systems deliver the same results.

At the end, one should note that this system cost is about 120 U.S. Dollars for its implementation, which is very affordable in order to be implemented in any car.

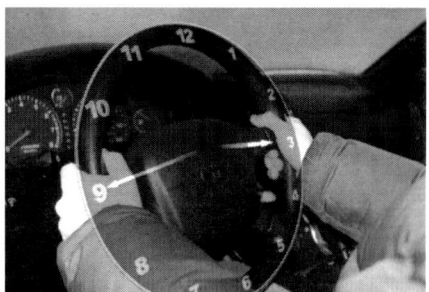 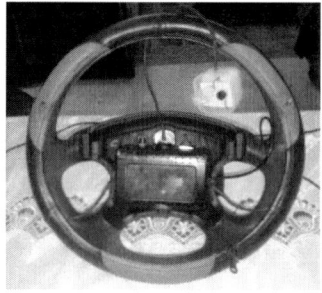

Figure 10. Positions of the MAX3010x sensors on the steering wheel.

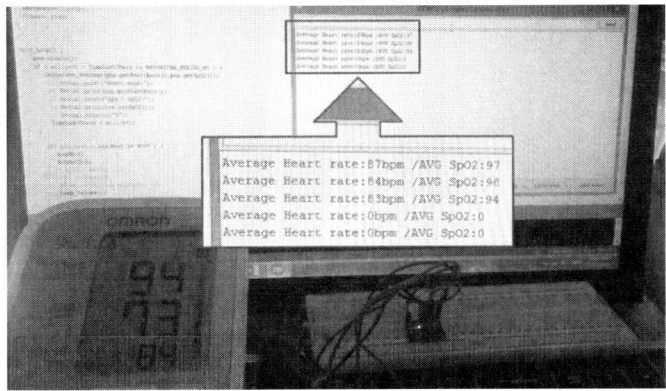

Figure 11. Comparing outputs from MAX30100 to NIBP machine.

7. CONCLUSION

This chapter has presented an embedded safety-related system, able to track the health of the driver and to signal any medical issue in case of occurrence. A phone application was developed with two main usages: the first is to monitor the user vital signs and to track its location whereas the other one is to signal a medical emergency to a health care provider.

The testing of this system has shown good results especially concerning the detection of emergency health problems, the communication between parties (the driver and the health care providers), the location sharing and the safe state testing.

As for the availability and reliability of this system, the design was made in such a way to allow its implementation in any car without the need to modify the electrical/electronic components. Added to that, the system switches off automatically when consecutive false alarms are generated.

As for the future works, we believe that this system has the potential to reach a global market of health care, as well as help decrease risk of death due to medical emergencies while driving, We see this device as the beginning of a larger project for improving health care. The proposed device may be developed further through the below proposed measures:

- Developing a server dedicated to the application thus all vitals will be saved so the user could retrieve them when needed;
- Adding more alarming systems and sensors;
- Adding more sensor used while driving for the protection of driver such as glucose and sleep detection sensor;
- Achieving more ranged testing to do all necessary calibration;
- Adopting the system by car manufactured to implement the system in cars for an emergency break or to safely park the car when driver is a bad state;
- Designing a system with lower electrical consumption and smaller size to be easily implemented in any car;
- Applying and evaluating safety and reliability measures to enhance the dependability of the system according to safety standards, which will be an essential part of the final target application.

REFERENCES

[1] U.S. Department of Transportation, "*Traffic Safety Facts*," NHTSA, Washington, 2009.

[2] U.S. Department of Transportation, "*The Contribution of Medical Conditions to Passenger Vehicle Crashes*," NHTSA, Washington, 2009.

[3] Janani, N; Saranya, N. "Driver safety awareness and assistance system for cognitive vehicle control," in *IEEE International Conference on Advanced Communications, Control and Computing Technologies*, Ramanathapuram, India, 2014.

[4] Strickland, E. "Thus, based on the numbers obtained in Table 1, the main idea of the project was to develop a monitoring system able to detect abnormalities in some vital signs in such an easy way that does not confuse the driver while driving and force him indirectly to," *IEEE Spectrum*, 2017.

[5] English, A. "Cars that can monitor your health," *The Telegraph*, 2013.

[6] Talib, B; Mohammad, M; Zgallai, W. "Elderly condition monitoring and alert system," in *Advances in Science and Engineering Technology International Conferences (ASET)*, Abu Dhabi, 2018.

[7] Constant, N; Douglas-Prawl, O; Johnson, S; Mankodiya, K. "Pulse-Glasses: An Unobtrusive, Wearable HR Monitor with Internet-of-Things Functionalities," in *IEEE 12th International Conference on Wearable and Implantable Body Sensor Networks (BSN)*, Cambridge, 2015.

[8] Chandrasekhar, A; Kim, CS; Naji, M; Natarajan, K; Hahn, JO; Mukkamala, R. "Smartphone-based blood pressure monitoring via the oscillometric finger-pressing method," *Science Translational Medicine*, vol. 10, pp. 1-11, 2018.

[9] Narendra Swaroop, K; Chandu, K; Gorrepotu, R; Deb, S. "A health monitoring system for vital signs using IoT," *Internet of Things*, vol. 5, pp. 116-129, 2019.

[10] Tay, F; Guo, D; Xu, L; Nyan, M; Yap, K. "MEMSWear-biomonitoring system for remote vital signs monitoring," *Journal of the Franklin Institute*, vol. 346, no. 6, pp. 531-542, 2009.

[11] Klingeberg, T; Schilling, M. "Mobile wearable device for long term monitoring of vital signs," *Computer Methods and Programs in Biomedicine*, vol. 106, no. 2, pp. 89-96, 2012.

[12] Jung, SJ; Shin, HS; Chung, WY. *"Highly sensitive driver health condition monitoring system using nonintrusive active electrodes,"* Elsevier B.V, pp. 691-698, 2012.

[13] Singh, R; Sarkar, A; Annop, C. "A health monitoring system using multiple non-contact ECG sensors for automotive drivers," in *IEEE International Instrumentation and Measurement Technology Conference*, Taipei, Taiwan, 2016.

[14] Lee, Y; Liu, S; Lin, H; Tseng, W. "Driver's health management system using nanosecond pulse near-field sensing technology," in *International Conference on Computer, Communications, and Control Technology (I4CT)*, Langkawi, Malaysia, 2014.

[15] Churpek, M; Adhikari, R; Edelson, D. "The value of vital sign trends for detecting clinical deterioration on the wards," *Resuscitation*, vol. 102, pp. 1-5, 2016.

[16] Maxim Integrated, "Pulse Oximeter and Heart-Rate Sensor IC for Wearable Health," Maxim Integrated Products, Inc, San Jose, 2014.

[17] Guangzhou, HC. "H-06 Product data sheet," Guangzhou HC Information Technology Co., Ltd., China, 2011.

[18] Walter, D; Sherman, M. Learning MIT App Inventor, Indiana: Pearson, 2014.

[19] Bottom Line, "Get with the times: You're driving all wrong," NBC News, 22 March 2012. [Online]. Available: https://www.nbcnews.com/businessmain/get-times-youre-driving-all-wrong-518710. [Accessed 10 April 2019].

[20] Ryan, T. "6 Road Rules You're Probably Breaking," CANSTAR, 5 May 2016. [Online]. Available: https://www.canstar.com.au/car-insurance/6-road-rules-youre-probably-breaking/. [Accessed 10 April 2019].

[21] Jakkar, R; Pahuja, R; Saini, R; Sahu, B. "Drunk-Driver Detection and Alert System (DDDAS) for Smart Vehicles," *American Journal of Traffic and Transportation Engineering*, vol. 2, no. 4, pp. 45-58, 2017.

[22] Driving tests, "Do You Hold a Steering Wheel Correctly? 3 Crucial Aspects of Safe Driving," *Driving tests*, 2019.

In: Vital Signs: An Overview
Editors: Roy Abi Zeid Daou et al.
ISBN: 978-1-53617-765-7
© 2020 Nova Science Publishers, Inc.

Chapter 6

STRUCTURAL AND FUNCTIONAL ABNORMALITIES IN MAJOR DEPRESSIVE DISORDER

Lara Hamawy[1], Ahmed Alnaggar[1], Khaled Omais[1], Mohamad Abou Ali[1], Mohamad Hajj-Hassan[1] and Abdallah Kassem[2,*]

[1]Department of Biomedical Engineering,
Lebanese International University, Lebanon
[2]ECCE Department, Faculty of Engineering,
Notre Dame University, Lebanon

ABSTRACT

Major Depressive Disorder (MDD), also known as clinical depression or unipolar depression, is a psychiatric disorder characterized by feelings of sadness that lead to physical and cognitive impairments. The nature of its symptomatology makes this disorder crippling, and patients are increasing worldwide. Moreover, MDD has huge costs on the

---

[*] Corresponding Author's Email: akassem@ndu.edu.lb.

community, as most of the patients cannot work for long periods of time. The World Health Organization estimated that MDD affects over 350 million people worldwide and is the leading source of disability and disease burden. In the current project, we conducted both morphometric analysis and functional connectivity analysis to investigate the underlying neural mechanisms of this disorder. We extracted the cortical volume and surface area from high-resolution MRI data of MDD patients and matched healthy controls. In order to investigate the functional correlations of the structural changes, we performed a seed-based functional connectivity analysis. Specifically, we extracted the regions showing significant differences in the structural analysis as regions of interest (ROI). Then, the time series of each ROI was extracted and correlated with each voxel of the cerebral cortex. Statistical analysis of the seed-based functional connectivity revealed significant decreases of functional connectivity between the seed region and the bilateral precuneus. The decreased functional connectivity in the mood-related regions might be caused by disorganization of the cortical architectures in these regions. In conclusion, the investigations of this research have reflected several differences between the healthy controls and MDD patients using structural analysis and functional connectivity analysis. Significant cortical volume and area reductions in the left middle frontal gyrus in MDD patients have been revealed as compared with healthy controls. The functional connectivity analysis showed significant functional connectivity decreases in the bilateral precuneus of MDD patients. Consequently, understanding the pathogenesis of MDD suggested contributing to developing effective therapy of this disease.

Keywords: major depressive disorder, depression, cortical volume, functional connectivity, structural connectivity

INTRODUCTION

Depression is a life-long situation in which periods of wellness alternate with recurrences of illness and may require long-term behavior to keep symptoms from returning, just like any other chronic medical illness [1]. Depression is a mood disorder that causes a persistent feeling of sadness and loss of interest. It is called major depressive disorder or clinical depression. It affects how patients feel, think and behave, and it can lead to a variety of emotional and physical problems. Patients have trouble in doing normal day-to-day activities and sometimes they may feel as if life isn't worth living. Unfortunately, depression may require long-term treatment [1]. Most people with depression feel better with medication, psychological counseling or both. Many efforts were made to treat depression, but up to 80% of patients are still affected [1]. Major depressive disorder (MDD) is characterized by abnormalities in both brain structure and function within the front limbic network. However, there is no much information known about the link between the structural and functional abnormalities in MDD. Here, we used a multimodal neuroimaging approach to investigate the relationship between structural connectivity and functional connectivity within the front limbic network. Mental illness in the United States is caused by depression affecting more than 19 million persons. Furthermore, 25% of women and 10% of men have one or more incidents of significant depression. That means such conditions require forms of interventions during lifetimes. Depression affects the lives of family and friends and society as it affects also the person who suffers from depression [2]. Figure 1 shows the lifetime incidence of depression in the United States estimated in 2005 according to the American Medical Association journal [3].

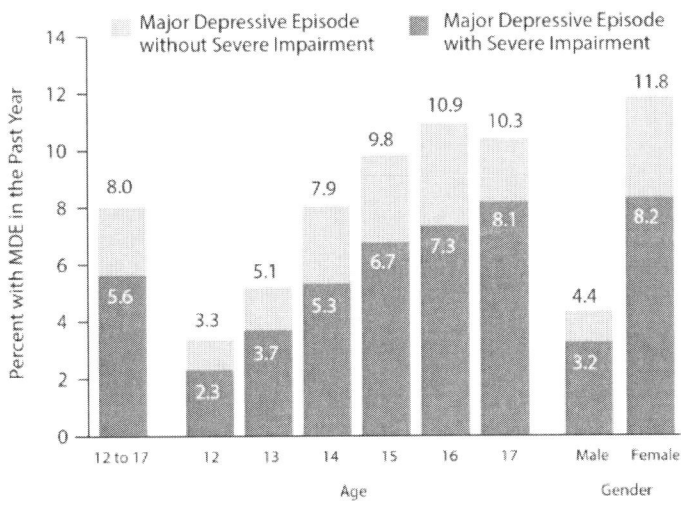

Figure 1. Lifetime incidence of depression in the United States estimated in 2005 according to American Medical Association journal [3].

LITERATURE REVIEW

Types of Depression

There are different types of depression. Symptoms can range from relatively minor to severe, so it is helpful to be aware of the conditions' ranges and their symptoms.

- Major Depressive Disorder is a considerable mental health situation described by repetitive and intense moods of unhappiness and desperation. The condition affects many parts of life, counting work, colleagues as well as relationships. It can also affect temper, manners and several physical roles, such as desire and sleep. People with MDD can also be characterized by loss of interest in daily activities. Occasionally, they may also sense as if life isn't worth living [4].
- Dysthymic Disorder is one of the most severe types of depression. People with Dysthymia describe their mood as sad or 'down in the dumps.' Dysthymia's person is characterized by having low self-esteem, an overall feeling of inadequacy, feeling of hopelessness and difficulty with productivity [4].
- Melancholic Depression is one type of major depressive disorder with melancholic features. Though this kind is considered to be seen as a different disorder, the American Psychiatric Association (APA) identified it as a distinct emotional disorder. In its place, melancholia is now measured as an indicator key for MDD [4].
- Psychotic Depression is the third type of depression. Individuals with such depressive form can lose touch with truth and knowledge. This can include hallucinations or delusions, such as believing that they are bad or evil, or that they are being examined. They can also be suspicious, feeling as though everyone is against them or that they are the cause of illness or bad actions occurring around them [4].

MAJOR DEPRESSIVE DISORDER SYMPTOMS

Gloom is a normal part of human practice. Individuals possibly will feel unhappy or depressed when a loved one dies or when they're surviving life-threatening problems, such as a split-up or severe illness. Yet, these moods are normally short-lived. When feelings of sadness extend for a long period of time then the person may face major depressive disorder. MDD is also referred as clinical depression that affects many areas of life. It disturbs temper and behavior as well as numerous bodily functions, such as desire and sleep. MDD individuals often miss the joy of activities and have worry about carrying out everyday activities. It is one of the greatest mutual mental illnesses in the United States. In 2015, closely 7 out of a hundred of Americans over age 18 had an experience of MDD. Some people with MDD never pursued treatment. However, the majority can be restored with the treatment. Medicines, psychoanalysis and other procedures can effectively treat people with MDD and help them manage their symptoms.

A mental health professional refers to the patient symptoms, feeling and behavior patterns in order to diagnose depression. Filling a questionnaire or answering to questions are parts of procedures used in diagnosis. Diagnostic and Statistical Manual of Mental Disorders (DSM) listed some symptoms criteria that must be respected to identify depression. The manuals aid medical experts analyze emotional health situations. According to its procedures, the patient must have 5 or more of the succeeding indications, and experienced them at least once a day for a period of more than 2 weeks [4]:

- You sense unhappy or short-tempered most of the day, nearly every day.
- You are fewer attentive in most actions you once liked.
- You unexpectedly loss or gain weight or have a change in desire.
- You have to worry about falling asleep or want to sleep more than normal.

- You experience feelings of impatience.
- You feel remarkably drained and have a lack of vitality.
- You feel valueless or guilty.
- You have trouble focusing, thinking, or making choices.
- You think about hurting yourself or killing yourself.

BRAIN STRUCTURE

There are three main parts of the human brain: cerebrum, cerebellum, and brainstem. Each of these three components has its different functions and characteristics, though the whole brain is highly cooperating with each other. The brain stem is under the cerebellum and connects the cerebrum spinal cord and cerebellum. This structure is accountable for the basic vital life functions such as maintaining consciousness, heartbeat, breath, blood pressure, digestion and regulating the sleep cycle. The cerebellum is located under cerebrum and behind brain stem. Cerebellum structure is associated with the functions of regulation and coordination of movement, posture, and balance.

The largest part of the human brain is cerebrum or cortical cortex, which is associated with higher brain functions such as thought and action; it is divided into left and right cerebral hemispheres. Both cerebral hemispheres are connected to a very large nerve bundle called corpus callosum. The cerebral cortex, shown in Figure 2, is segmented into four sections the frontal lobe, the parietal lobe, the occipital lobe, and the temporal lobe [5].

There are three types of brain elements that can be generally segmented into gray matter (GM), white matter (WM) and cerebrospinal fluid (CSF). Figure 3 shows a magnetic resonance imaging (MRI) with gray and white matter labeled [6]. Gray matter known as the cortex that consists of the nerves cells bodies and it is located in the exterior part of the brain. White matter is known as the medulla that transmits the electrical signals that carry the messages between neurons and it is located in the interior part of the brain. Cerebrospinal fluid is a transparent fluid that fills ventricles and surrounds the brain and spinal cord. Therefore, it can absorb the shock and keep the brain under protection [6].

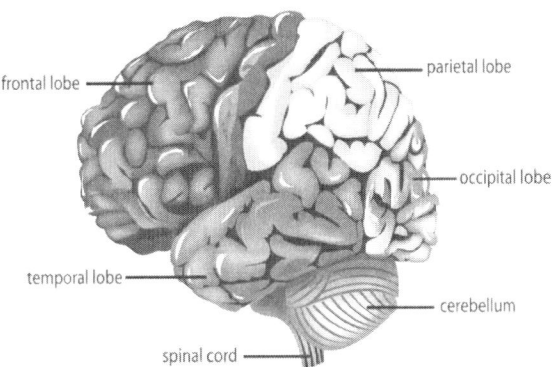

Figure 2. Part of the human brain [5].

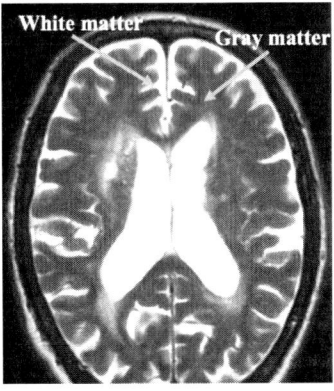

Figure 3. MRI image showing the gay matter and white matter in the brain [6].

Brain Connectivity

Brain connectivity has complex organization networks as shown in Figure 4. This complex network is not only documented segregation and integration during high progressions but also it can give clinical values of alterations encountered in development, aging, or neurological diseases. Recently, researchers describe brain networks as a small world and mathematical model, allowing the greatest efficiency with nominal energy and connecting cost [7].

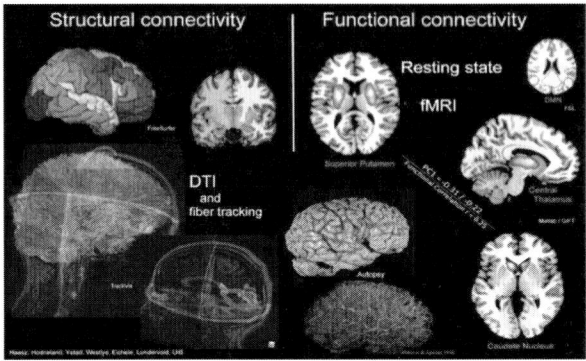

Figure 4. Structural and functional connectivity assessed with multimodal MRI [7].

Structural Connectivity

Structural connectivity is defined as the set of physical connections between neural units. In other words, anatomical connectivity is related to a complex of physical or structural (synaptic) connections that link sets of neurons or neuronal elements, as well as their connected structural biophysical features encapsulated in parameters such as synaptic strength or effectiveness. Actually, structural connections are impartially unchanging over short period scales (seconds or minutes). However, on larger period scales (days) they are subject to important morphological variations due to neuroplasticity. Neuroplasticity is the term that describes the changes in the individual's brain during stages of life. Thus, reaching 300 microns (1 micron = 10^{-6} meter) resolution of the human cortex that has been applied by the progression of the high-resolution MR. Such scales paved the road to reach the same resolution obtained by histological analysis. There are two different approaches to investigate structural connectivity. The first is to evaluate the correlation of diffusion parameters in predefined regions of interest (ROI) with either behavioral performance or with fMRI activation peaks observed for numerical tasks. Diffusion imaging utilizes the variability of "Brownian motion" of water molecules in brain tissue. Brownian motion refers to the random movement of molecules. Fractional anisotropy is a method that is used to emphasize and evaluate white matter fiber tract. This method has been applied to MRI scans in diffusion-weighted images. Diffusion-tensor imaging (DTI) is an MRI technique that uses fractional anisotropic diffusion to estimate the white matter organization of the brain. Fractional anisotropy (FA) and/or radial diffusion often used diffusion parameters in this analysis. The second approach is fiber tractography, which allows for the virtual reconstruction of the entire white matter pathway. Fiber tractography (FT) is a 3D reconstruction technique to access neural tracts using data collected by DTI [8, 9].

Functional Connectivity

In contrast, functional connectivity is a concept of statistics. Deviations are captured from statistical independence between spatially and distributed neuronal units. This statistical dependence is related to the estimation of covariance, spectral coherence or phase-locking. Functional brain areas can be detected by the means of their time-consuming variations in signal strength. The stream synchrony of blood can be identified in sensorimotor areas, language regions, and the visual cortex by fMRI. Regions that are triggered by the motor, language or visual tasks are characterized by slow synchronous fluctuations. The normal mammalian brain, performing no tasks, is characterized by the slow fluctuations of cerebral blood flow. These fluctuations in the functionally interconnected areas of the brain are synchronous even if the related regions are separated by a considerable distance. The synchrony of the blood flow fluctuations in functionally related brain regions implies the existence of neuronal connections that facilitate the coordinated activity. The term functional connectivity is used to describe the interdependence of the functionally related brain regions. Functional connectivity can be studied using electrodes positioned in the brain, radioisotopes administered intravenously and EEG. Thus, MRI added a new technique for studying such connectivity. Synchronous changes in the blood-oxygen-level-dependent (BOLD) can be reached by having high correlated fluctuations in signal intensity. fMRI uses rapidly acquired images to plot the place of enlarged bloodstream when an external stimulus is applied and detected. In fMRI, the signal amplitude or the signal intensity fluctuates temporally correlated with the performance of a task. This is recognized by the hemodynamic change localization resulting from the stimulus [10].

Functional Magnetic Resonance (fMRI)

Functional magnetic resonance imaging (fMRI) is a relatively new imaging technique that is used to map more complex functions e.g., emotions, face recognition, complex motor control, specialized language functions, etc... Figure 5 shows an example of a network for supporting resting-state fMRI related studies. Changes in blood oxygenation level in specific regions in the brain can be taken as a sign of activity in this region. Therefore, fMRI can be used to measure the difference of the magnetic field between the periods of the brain activation and rest states [11, 12].

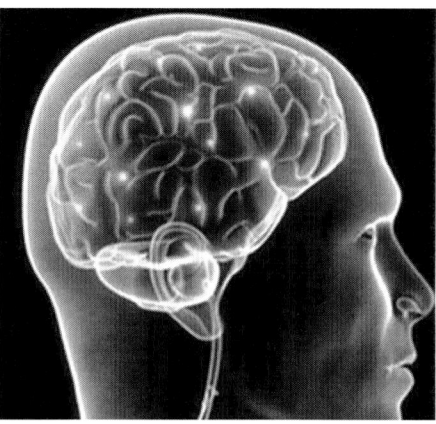

Figure 5. A network for supporting resting-state fMRI related studies [12].

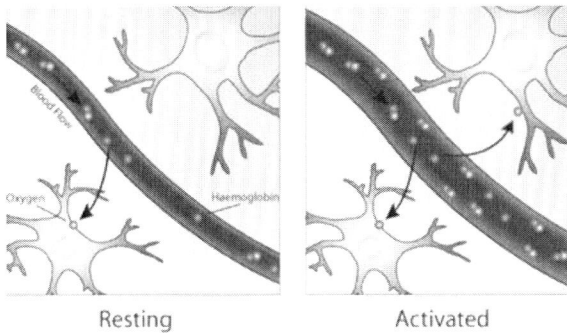

Figure 6. Direction of oxygenation change with increased activity [16].

Some functions in the cortical area may give some information about some psychological diseases such as depression. In addition, studying functional integration among segregated brain areas could reveal new insights regarding brain functionality and hierarchy [13].

In order to obtain fMRI images, there are many functional integration methods such as functional brain connectivity, for example, "Seed-based Correlation Analysis (SCA)." SCA is a common method to detect the functional connectivity in the brain. Based on regions of interest (ROI), connectivity is calculated as the correlation of time series for all other voxels in the brain. The result of this method is a connectivity map showing Z-scores for each voxel and how well its time series correlates with the time series of the seed [14]. Another method depends on component analysis individually. It is a technique used to suggest some hidden factors that underlie sets of random variables, signals, or measurements. It is called "Statistical and Computational Analysis." It gives a large database "samples" by defining a generative model for the observed multivariate data [15]; it has been developed to estimate the functional integration of spatially remote brain regions. Both conventional events related potential and time-frequency analysis may be used for this purpose.

Neuroimaging techniques have played an important role in exploring human brain especially fMRI. Instigation of brain areas needs energy which is provided by intake of fresh blood. For instance, a result activated area contains more blood circulation than the others and have different magnetic properties as shown in Figure 6. The difference can be observed by a strong permanent magnet, a gradient field magnet; a magnet with variable magnetic field and radio frequency (RF) transceivers inside the fMRI machine.

Problem Statement and Objectives

In general, there is no laboratory test that can detect the MDD or depression. Moreover, the MRI brain image does not reveal the MDD disease during diagnosis. When the MDD is not detected at an early stage it can negatively affect the patient's personal life, as well as sleeping, eating habits, and general health. 2 to 7% of adults with major depression die by committing suicide, and up to 60% of people who die by suicide had depression or another mood disorder. The diagnosis of major depressive disorder is based on the person's reported experiences and a mental status examination. It is unclear whether medications affect the risk of suicide. Major depressive disorder affected approximately 216 million persons (3% of the world's population) in 2015 [17]. It became the second most rated disease after the low back pain.

For all these reasons above, this proposed system is dedicated to assist people who suffer from depression by finding a technique that can detect early stages of depression using MRI technology.

In this research, the structural and functional connectivity of the cortical volume and surface area will be analyzed on 18 MDD patients. MRI images are used to analyze the structural connectivity of the brain region and fMRI is used to analyze the functional connectivity in the brain region [18, 19, 20]. Thus, the MDD disease will be detected by finding the relation between structural and functional connectivity and by comparing the results with healthy subjects.

METHODOLOGY

Finding a result for depressed people requires a study of the brain connection and brain structure. Recently, researches focused on a specific region and studied the functional connectivity within them instead of the whole-brain. During the cognitive and the emotional task paradigms, abnormal functional connectivity was shown in some region of interested of depressed patients. The first part of the methodology will cover the "Structural Analysis" of MDD and the second part is about the "Functional Analysis" of MDD.

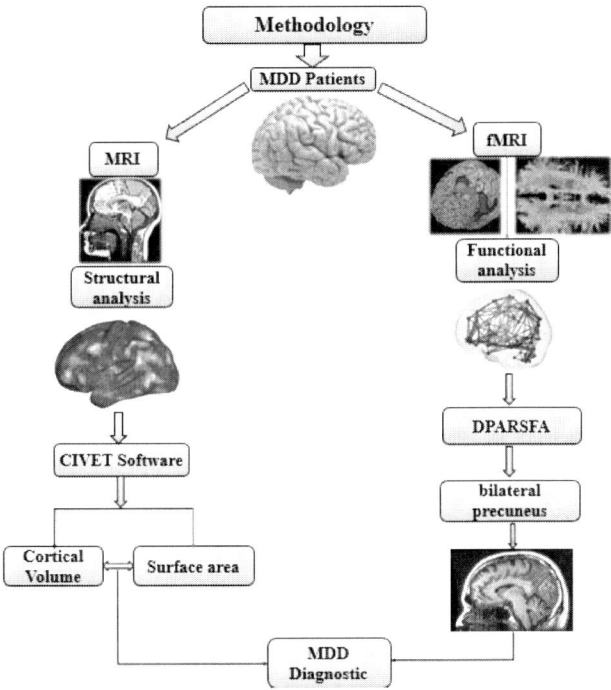

Figure 7. Block Diagram showing the Class Diagram and the following steps of the proposed system.

"Surface-Based Analysis" technique has been applied in our system; it is a group of brain morphometric techniques used to construct and analyze surfaces that represent structural boundaries within the brain. The advantage of the surface-based morphometry technique comes from high capability in detecting focal morphological changes based on an automated surface-based morphometry approach [21, 22]. Moreover, research has proved that surface-based method is more efficient than the volume-based brain mapping because it offers the structural characteristics of the brain, like surface change, complexity and change patterns in the brain during disease. MATLAB, SPM, CIVET and, DPARSFA software is employed in "Surface-based analysis" of the block diagram of the proposed system as shown in Figure 7.

Requirements and Specification Analysis

1) Subjects

Data has been collected from the outpatient clinic at Xuanwu Hospital in China. A total of 36 candidates take part in this analysis. 18 patients (4 men and 14 women) have medication-naïve with the first major depressive episode and 18 subjects are healthy. All candidates are treated according to the knowledgeable agreement form approved by Xuanwu Hospital Medical Research Ethics Group. The patients have been chosen according to the following criteria:

- Never used any "Psychotherapy" before created the assessment.
- Between eighteen and sixty years old.
- Never used the drugs.
- First-degree relatives should not have any of major psychiatric or neurological illness.
- The patient should not use any prescription.
- The patient has to agree to undergo a magnetic resonance imaging (MRI).
- Moreover, the patients who have any one of the following criteria will be removed from the list:
- If the patient suicided.
- Loss of realization, produced by pregnancy, breastfeeding during the trauma.

2) Clinical data

Table 1 depicts the clinical data used in the analysis of the 36 candidates.

Table 1. Clinical Data

	MDD patient	Healthy subject	P Value
Number of Subject	18	18	-
Gender (male/female)	4	14	-
Ages/Years	39.8 ± 9.3	39.0 ± 10.7	-
Disease duration/Years	6.7 ± 3.9	-	-
Hamilton Depression Rating Scale (HDRS)	(17.8 ± 3.6)	18 demographically	-

Image Acquisition

Collecting Data from MRI machine requires some steps in the anatomical and functional as follow:

1) Structural Image Acquisition

Three-T Siemens Tim Trio MRI was used to obtain 3-dimensional structural images. The parameter of the image was: TE (Echo Time) = 2.52ms, TR (Repetition Time) = 1900 ms, IT (Inversion Time) = 900 s, flip angle =9°, width = 1.0 mm, matrix =256 × 256, no gap, 176 slices, and voxel size =1×1 × 1mm.

2) Functional Image Acquisition

MRI configured in BOLD signal levels, an echo planar imaging is used to obtain the images and the settings were as follow:

TE = 30ms, TR = 2000ms, Matrix: 64×64, Flip angle: 90°, Thickness slice: 3 mm, Field of view: 220×220, Gap slice: 1 mm, and Voxel size = 3.4×3.4×4mm^3). During fMRI, all patients were instructed to minimize their movement as much as possible, relax, stop thinking, and keep their eyes closed.

Data Pre-Processing

Data pre-processing contains an anatomical and functional analysis before giving the final result. The data-preprocessing steps are shown in Figure 8. Figure 9 lists the pre-processing steps that are performed in SPM (Statistical Parametric Mapping).

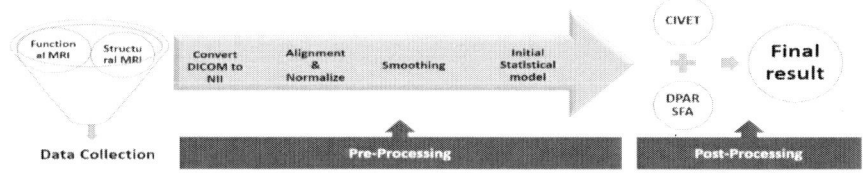

Figure 8. Data Processing.

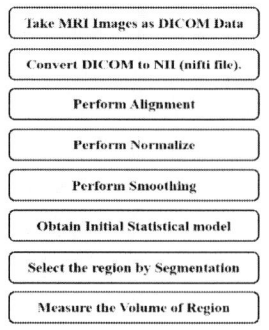

Figure 9. Pre-processing steps.

SPM (Statistical Parametric Mapping) is a program launched by associates & traitors of the Wellcome Trust Centre for Neuroimaging in the UK, to facilitate the processing of the MRI data for the hypothesis of the neuroimaging researchers. It is used for analysis of brain imaging data sequences by using time-series or different series. SPM has a different type of extension called NII (nifti file). Thus, the MRI images should be converted from DICOM to the NII type. The general steps will be discussed and for more information you can see the SPM manual, from this website (http://www.fil.ion.ucl.ac.uk/spm/):

- Download the SPM files from the above link and connect it with MATLAB as Path and sub path.
- After receiving MRI data from the research center, all images are converted to NII files by using DICOM Import.
- Alignment is applied to the images in order to remove the noise and to put all data with the same movement and rotation.
- Normalization and smoothing are also applied to the images to give a clear result and to apply the specific processing for the ROI.

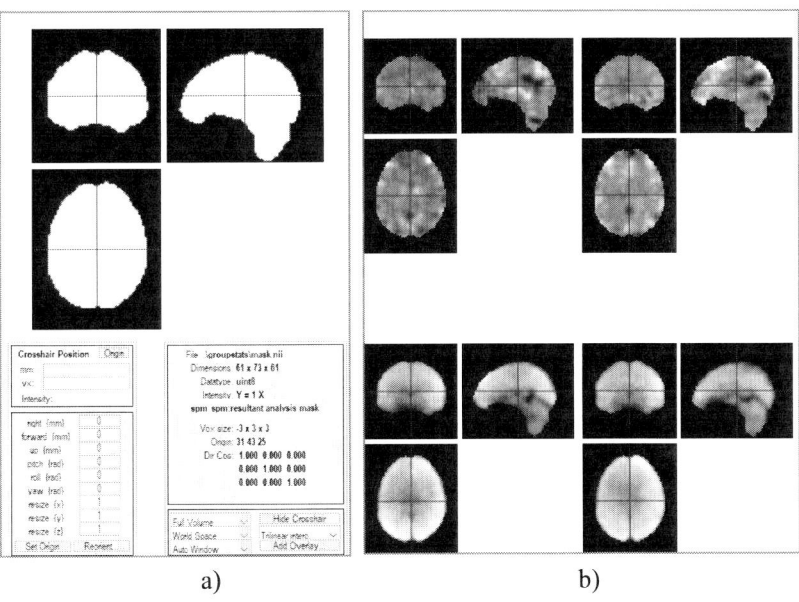

Figure 10. a) Mask used to the model of statistical analysis; b) Beta image for MDD and HC in model of statistical analysis.

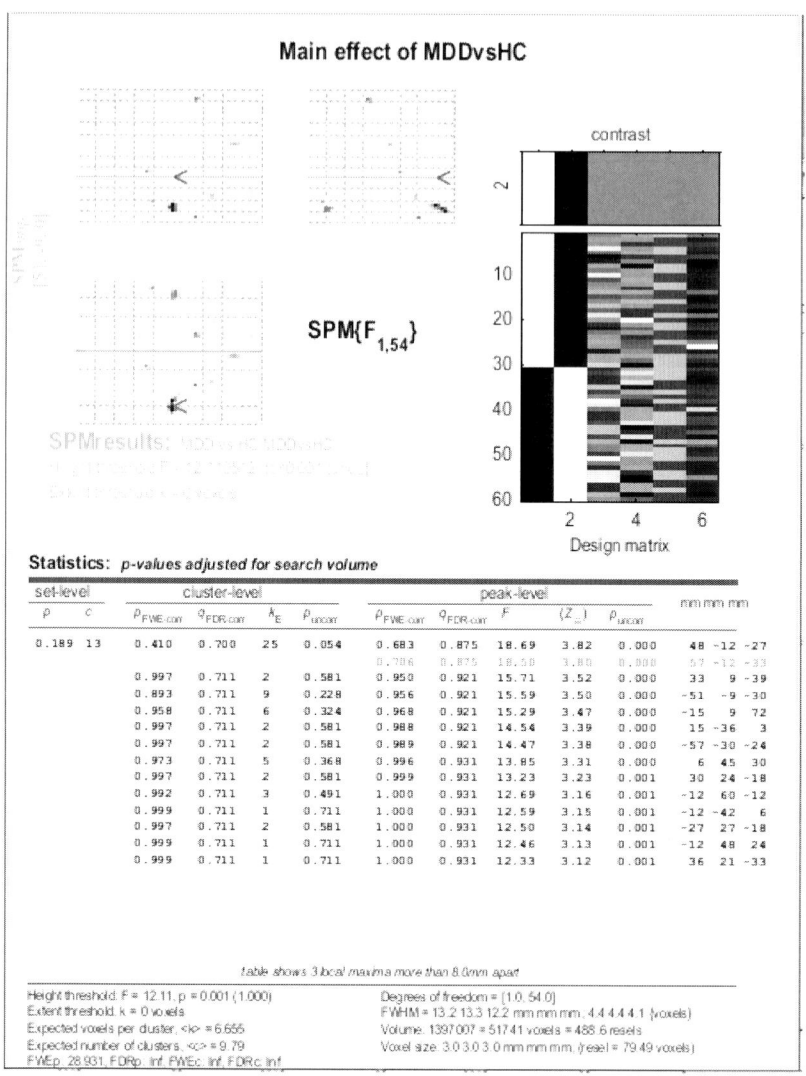

Figure 11. Adding a contrast to show the Difference of two Statistical Model.

- Image segmentation classified the data of each subject into different types of tissue. The separation is defined according to tissue specification maps and to the probability to find the tissue type at a specific location. Typically, the separation of tissue was prepared to get a gray matter, white matter, CSF bone, soft tissue, and air/background (if using TPM/TPMni).

- Initial Statistical Model to start the processing of functional and Structural MRI Data: The Statistical Model means that the Data of HC (Healthy Control) and MDD will be separated into two different groups. This separation will facilitate the processing to find the abnormalities. After that, the Mask will be applied for both groups of data in order to sum all MDD as one image and all HC as one image as shown in Figure 10 (a). Moreover, the beta image of every model will appear as shown in Figure 10 (b).

After image preprocessing, the abnormalities can appear if the contrast is added to the different groups by using the SPM as shown in Figure 11. Furthermore, the result from CIVET, DPARSFA will be discussed in the next paragraph.

By applying these preprocessing steps such as realignment, smoothing, and segmentation, data is collected in two groups in the statistical model. The first group is used for MDD data and the second for the HC (Healthy Control) data where each group is saved in a new file. Consequently, for any future processing just calling or loading these groups is applicable even in other programs.

Data Post-Processing

1) Processing of Structural MRI Data Using CIVET

All T1-weighted images (also referred to as T1WI or the "spin-lattice" relaxation time) is one of the basic pulse sequences in MRI and demonstrates differences in the T1 relaxation times of tissues. were processed by CIVET software. First of all, registration with the CIVET program using MNI152 standard space (MNI stands for the Montreal Neurological Institute of McGill University Health Center) has been applied. Then, some corrections for images like normalization and alignments are performed. Next, anatomical images segmentation was applied to get the white matter (WM), gray matter (GM) and background via an advanced neural net classifier in order to assist the estimation of the partial volume for each voxel of the brain. Then, the anatomical segmentation is applied by using constrained Laplacian-based to generate (outer) vertex-wise surface meshes of gray matter and the (inner) surfaces which is white matter by hemisphere. Finally, the volume in the middle of the cortical surface which located at the symmetrical midpoint between the internal and external surface (40.962 vertexes in each hemisphere) was calculated.

2) Functional Connectivity Analysis Using DPARSFA

DPARSFA program was used in processing all-functional MRI data. In order to do magnetization equilibrium, the initial 10 Measurements of each scan were rejected. The pre-processing involved are:

- Slice timing.
- Head motion alteration.
- Normalizing to the MNI model.
- Re-sampling $3\times3\times3mm^3$.
- Smoothing via 4mm Gaussian kernel to reduction longitudinal noise.
- Sequential band pass filtering.
- Relapsing out irritation indications including head motion constraints, white matter, and cerebrospinal fluid.

The ROI (region of interest) are extracted in the cortical volume in order to find the difference between groups. Average time series of the seed ROI was calculated for individual subject. After that, correlation coefficients are estimated among the mean time series of the ROI and all the voxels through the total brain. Then, this correlation factor is transformed to z value via (Fisher's r-to-z transformation) to improve their normality.

IMPLEMENTATION

As mentioned, this study is divided into two parts. The first one was studying the structural connectivity and the second was studying the functional connectivity of the brain. The aim of this research was reached by taking into consideration variable methods to get information about specific regions of interest starting with SPM, CIVET, and DPARSF.

Structural Statistical Analysis

In every point across all subjects in MNI (Montreal Neurological Institute) space, the statistical analysis was achieved to find the group variances between patients with MDD and Healthy Subjects. The applied statistical model is the general linear model (GLM) for both cortical volume and surface area measurements in MDD patients and normal controls. Then, a corrected P value was obtained for multiple comparisons using random field theory [23]. The level of significance for clusters was set at P value of less than 0.05 after multiple comparison corrections.

Functional Statistical Analysis

In order to study the functional connectivity of both groups, the Seed-based Correlation Analysis (SCA) has been conducted using DPARSF software. Then, a corrected cluster-wise P value was obtained for each cluster using Gaussian random field theory. The level of significance was set at $P < 0.05$ after correction for multiple comparisons.

RESULTS AND DISCUSSION

Structural Results

Compared with healthy controls, we found a significant reduction in the left middle frontal of the cortical volume (see Figure 12). Also, significant reductions of surface area in the left middle frontal gyrus in patients with MDD have been observed (see Figure 13).

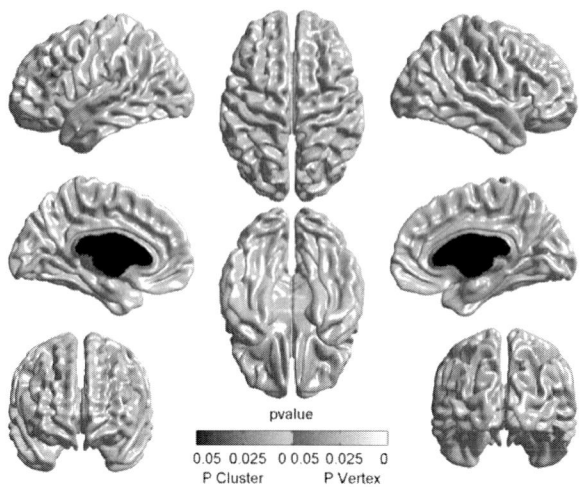

Figure 12. Significant cortical volume; the results were corrected for multiple comparisons (P < 0.05).

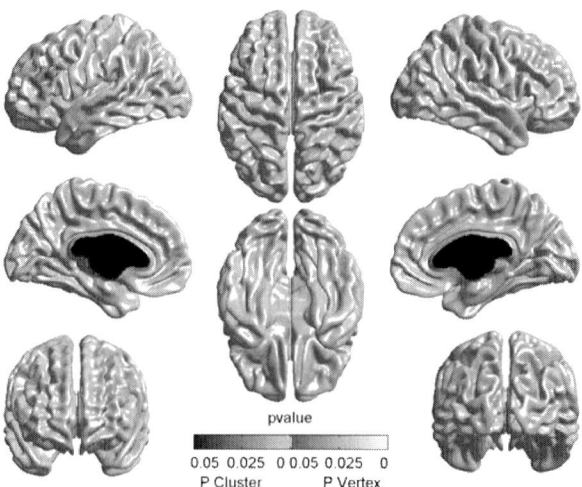

Figure 13. P-cluster and P vertex in the surface area showing the difference between the cortical volume and surface area in the structural imaging.

Discussion

The structural analysis of both MDD patients and the matched healthy controls showed that patients with depression have significant reductions in the left middle frontal gyrus of both cortical volume and area. In figures 12 and 13 the blue and orange points describe the difference in structural abnormalities and the concentration of the color depending on the variance of change. Furthermore, we can observe in the different brain orientation regions, the frontal lobe is the most active, where the middle frontal gyrus is located. The functions of the frontal lobe are:

- Defining the good from bad along through the moments of activities.
- Long-standing memory.
- Sensitive occupations.
- Person's characters and mood.

Nonetheless, it is hard to precisely define any specific section of the brain in terms of functionality. Moreover, the frontal cortex in the brain of humans has numerous areas; one of them is called Brodmann Area 9 (BA9). This area lies in both hemispheres and intricate in temporary memory [24]. The left part of the hemisphere is responsible for empathy, processing a pleasant and unpleasant emotional sequence and reaction to the negative emotions [25, 26]. Furthermore, there is another area of the frontal cortex called Brodmann area 46 (BA46); it is known as middle frontal area 46 and it plays a role in working and attention memory [27].

Cortical volume is confounded by two genetically and evolutionarily distinct properties, which are cortical width and surface area [28, 29]. A study held by Kyu-Man Han mentioned the changes in cortical thickness, cortical and subcortical volume and white matter veracity among first episode, medication-naïve MDD patients and healthy subjects by using an automatic process of Free Surfer and Tract-based spatial data (TBSS) to study among the areas [30]. The patients who are suffering from the first episode MDD showed meaningfully reduced cortical volume in the caudal frontal cingulated gyrus when the threshold was P < 0.0015. Also, this experimental study changed white matter integrity in the body of the corpus callosum P < 0.01 which exposed to the reduced cortical volume of the caudal middle frontal gyrus and medial orbitofrontal gyrus. Another study mentioned in [30] used VBM-DARTEL to investigate together cortical width and surface area in the first episode, treatment-naïve and mid-life MDD that proposed to explain the main pathophysiology of this illness and its premature effect on the brain. Its experiential increases in cortical thickness of rostral middle frontal gyrus and other brain regions correlate with our study and prove the accuracy of our system's results. We can study the cortical volume by two genetically and evolutionarily distinct properties, which are cortical width and surface area [28, 29]. There are large number of studies done on the cortical thickness and surface area and prove the same results as we get in Figures 12 and 13. The colored areas represent a biomarker of early detection of the MDD.

Functional Results

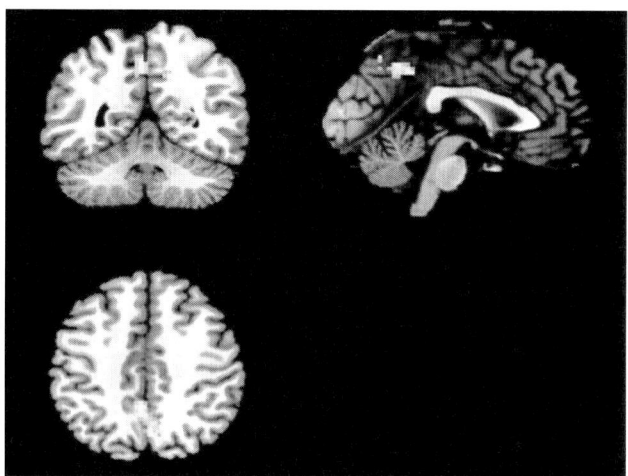

Figure 14. Brain areas display meaningfully reduced functional connectivity in the bilateral precuneus. The outcomes were modified for numerous judgments (P < 0.05 RFT-corrected).

Related to healthy controls and MDD patients, the statistical analysis of the seed-based functional connectivity revealed significant decreases of functional connectivity between the seed area and the bilateral precuneus in MDD patients as shown in Figure 14.

Discussion

The most common aspects reveal an overall perspective on structural and functional abnormalities in MDD patients are cortical volume, surface area, and functional connectivity. Any changes of the functional connectivity in the areas that are linked to the attitude may lead to MDD or any type of depression.

In summary, the investigations of this research have reflected several variations between the healthy subjects and MDD patients using structural and functional analysis. Reduction in the left middle frontal cortex, reductions of functional connectivity among the seed area and the bilateral precuneus were meaningfully presented. This proposed system can be used to confirm the clinical perceptions of the depression severity in the patients. It also proposes that the abnormalities in this area could be an accurate indicator of MDD, in which, it will be proved in further future studies. Moreover, studying the disorder-precise organic structures recommended shiny brain growing trails and mechanisms, like cortical volume and surface area, which would assist in the growth of consistent investigation in MDD.

CONCLUSION AND FUTURE WORKS

Major depressive disorder (MDD) is related to irregularities in cortical and subcortical brain constructions also to problems in their connectivity. This study investigates the difference between depressed people and healthy control spotting the light on the cortical volume and area reduction in the left middle frontal gyrus. After analysis, results showed that there is a significant reduction in the gray matter volume in cortical volume and reductions in the left middle frontal gyrus.

These variations in first-episode, treatment-naïve, and mid-life MDD patients might mirror a dynamic disease-related cortical alteration near to disease start, and consequently possibly offer significant new vision into the early neurobiology of the illness.

More studies are needed in order to understand the mechanism of the abnormalities in MDD. However, the diagnoses of this disease are still very vague for researchers that are trying to find new solutions. May some techniques and/or methods can be used such as, the correlation methods. Moreover, machine learning can be added to the new generations of MRI as a tool. This field needs a lot of research to make a real distinction in the "Depression Diagnostic."

ACKNOWLEDGMENTS

The authors would like to thank Dr. Ahmed Ameen for providing the MRI images.

REFERENCES

[1] Ye, M. et al. (2015). "Changes of Functional Brain Networks in Major Depressive Disorder: A Graph Theoretical Analysis of Resting-State fMRI," *POLS,* vol. 10 (9).

[2] "*depressionclinic,*" 12 May 2013. [Online]. Available: http://www.depressionclinic.com/mentalhealth/depression/causeetiology/default.htm. [Accessed 16 Nov 2017].

[3] Lieber, A., "*Major Depression (Unipolar Depression),*" 10 Jul 2017. [Online]. Available: https://www.psycom.net/depression.central.major.html. [Accessed 28 Nov 2017].

[4] Kerr, M., "Major Depressive Disorder (Clinical Depression)," *health line*, 27 June 2017. [Online]. Available: https://www.healthline.com/health/clinical-depression#Overview1. [Accessed 28 Nov 2018].

[5] "*parts-of-the-human-brain*," 1 Mar 2012. [Online]. Available: http://www.humanbrainfacts.org/parts-of-the-human-brain.php. [Accessed 17 Nov 2018].

[6] Monnig, M., "The Brains of Addicts," *MentalHelp*, 1 Apr. 2016. https://www.mentalhelp.net/addiction/the-brains-of-addicts/ [Accessed 17 Nov 2018].

[7] Guye, M., Bartolomei, F., Ranjeva, J.P. (2008). "Imaging structural and functional connectivity: towards a unified definition of human brain organization?" *Current Opinion in Neurology*, 21(4), pp. 393–403.

[8] Parker, G. P. (2004). "Analysis of MR diffusion weighted images," *British Institute of Radiology*, vol. 77, no. 2, p. 107-185.

[9] O'Donnell, L. J., et al. (2006). "A Method for Clustering White Matter Fiber Tracts," AJ*NR Am J Neuroradio*l. 27(5), 1032–1036.

[10] Cordes, D. et al. (2000). "Mapping Functionally Related Regions of Brain with Functional Connectivity MR Imaging," *American Journal of Neuroradiology*, vol. (9), pp. 1636-1644.

[11] Devlin, H. "*What is Functional Magnetic Resonance Imaging (fMRI)?*" psychcentral, 1 Jun 2016. [Online]. Available: https://psychcentral.com/lib/what-is-functional-magnetic-resonance-imaging-fmri/. [Accessed 3 Nov 2018].

[12] Yan, C.G., "The R-fMRI Network –a network for supporting resting-state fMRI related Studies," *The R-fMRI Network*, 1 Jun 2014. [Online]. Available: http://rfmri.org/. [Accessed 17 Nov 2018].

[13] Friston, K. J. (2011). "Functional and effective connectivity: a review," *Brain Connectivity*, 1(1), pp. 13-36.

[14] C-PAC 1.5.0 Beta Documentation, "*Seed-based Correlation Analysis (SCA) and Dual Regression,*" Mar 2010. [Online]. Available: https://fcp-indi.github.io/docs/user/sca.html#seed-based-correlation-analysis-sca-and-dual-regression. [Accessed 4 Nov 2018].

[15] Hyvärinen, Aapo, et al. (2001). *Independent Component Analysis*, A Wiley-Interscience Publication, NY.
[16] Devlin, H. (2018). "What is Functional Magnetic Resonance Imaging (fMRI)?" Department of Clinical Neurology, University of Oxford, https://psychcentral.com/lib/what-is-functional-magnetic-resonance-imaging-fmri/ [Accessed 17 Nov 2018].
[17] Vos, T., et al. (2016). "Global, regional, and national incidence, prevalence, and years lived with disability for 310 diseases and injuries, 1990–2015: a systematic analysis for the Global Burden of Disease Study 2015," *Lancet*, London, 388(10053), pp. 1545-1602.
[18] Wang, F., et al. (2009). "Functional and Structural Connectivity Between the Perigenual Anterior Cingulate and Amygdala in Bipolar Disorder," *Biological Psych*iatry, 66(5), pp. 516-521.
[19] Smagula S. F., Aizenstein H. J. (2016). "Brain structural connectivity in late-life major depressive disorder," *Biological Psychiatry Cognitive Neuroscience Neuroimaging*, 1(3), pp. 271-277.
[20] Fang, P., et al. (2012). "Increased Cortical-Limbic Anatomical Network Connectivity in Major Depression Revealed by Diffusion Tensor Imaging," *PLoS One,* 7(9).
[21] White, T., et al. (2018). "Automated quality assessment of structural magnetic resonance images in children: Comparison with visual inspection and surface based reconstruction," *Human Brain Mapping banner,* 39(3), pp. 1218-1231.
[22] West, J., et al. (2012). "Novel whole brain segmentation and volume estimation using quantitative MRI," *European Radiology*, 22(5), pp. 998–1007.
[23] Hayasaka, S., et al. (2004). "Nonstationary cluster-size inference with random field and permutation methods," *Neuroimage*, 22(2), pp. 676-687.
[24] Babiloni, C., et al. (2001). "Human cortical responses during one-bit delayed-response tasks: an fMRI study," *Brain Research Bulletin*, 65(5), 2005.
[25] Farrow, T. F., et al, "Investigating the functional anatomy of empathy and forgiveness.," *Neuroreport*, 12(11), pp. 2433-2438.

[26] Lane, R. D., et al. (1997). "Neuroanatomical correlates of pleasant and unpleasant emotion.," *Neuropsychologia*, 35(11), pp. 1437-1444.
[27] Kerestes, R., et al. (2012). "Abnormal prefrontal activity subserving attentional control of emotion in remitted depressed patients during a working memory task with emotional distracters.," *Psychological Medicine*, 42(1), pp. 29-40.
[28] Panizzon, M. S., et al. (2009). "Distinct genetic influences on cortical surface area and cortical thickness.," *Cerebral Cortex*, 19(11), pp. 2728-2735.
[29] Hutton, C., et al. (2009). "A comparison between voxel-based cortical thickness and voxel-based morphometry in normal aging.," *Neuroimage*, 48(2), pp. 371-380.
[30] Han, K. M., et al. (2014). "Cortical thickness, cortical and subcortical volume, and white matter integrity in patients with their first episode of major depression.," *Journal of Affective Disorders*, vol. 155, pp. 42-48.

ABOUT THE EDITORS

Roy Abi Zeid Daou
Chairperson of Biomedical Technologies Department
Lebanese German University, Jounieh, Lebanon

Roy Abi Zeid Daou was born in Lebanon in September 29th, 1984. He obtained his engineering degree in robotics in 2007, his masters in 2008 and his Ph.D. degree in Control Systems in 2011. Actually, he is an associate professor in the Lebanese German University and the head of the Biomedical Technologies Department. His research focuses on fractional differentiation and its applications in physics domains, mainly in the hydropneumatic, diffusive interfaces, electrical, acoustic and seismic domains. He also working on the design, implementation and validation of safe system applied, mainly, to the biomedical domain.

Josef Börcsök
Chairperson of Computer Architecture and System
Programming Department
University of Kassel, Kassel, Germany

Josef BÖRCSÖK: He was born in 1959. He received his B.Sc. degree in 1986 (University of Applied Sciences in Darmstadt), the M.Sc. degree in

1991 (University of Kassel) and the Ph.D. in 1995 (Technical University of Ilmenau). He was for more than 10 years researchers in leading positions in the industry (Avionics, Industrial control and Safety-Computer). During this time he lectures at universities, as well as at universities of applied sciences with lectures of automation systems, computer technology, real-time systems, network techniques and safety-related computer technology. Since 2005 he is Professor and head of the Department Computer architecture and System programming at the University of Kassel in Germany.

INDEX

A

accelerometers, 28, 32, 37, 42, 46, 47, 52, 67, 75, 76
access, 139
activity level, 11
adolescents, 3
adrenal gland, 16
adults, ix, 2, 3, 6, 7, 8, 10, 11, 13, 142
aerobic capacity, 4, 9
aerobic exercise, 5, 6, 8, 12
age, 2, 3, 13, 17, 56, 98, 101, 135
aldosterone, 17
alertness, 3, 19
algorithm, 32, 35, 36, 41, 42, 48, 51, 52, 53, 69, 72, 74, 75
alveoli, 23
American Psychiatric Association, 134
amplitude, 36, 113, 140
anatomy, 158
anesthetics, 20, 21
anesthetization, 21
angiography, 24
anisotropy, 139

antidiuretic hormone, 17
anxiety, 18, 19, 20, 21, 29, 30
apnea, 20
appetite, 16
artificial intelligence, x, 33
Artificial Neural Networks, 28, 36, 37
aseptic, 24
aspiration, 23
assessment, 71, 84, 144, 158
atelectasis, 23
automation, 82, 83, 86, 104, 106, 162
automotive application, 118
automotive applications, 118
awareness, 29, 128

B

back pain, 142
Bangladesh, 70
barometric pressure, 43
base, x, 89
behaviors, 17
benefits, 1, 2, 3, 4, 87, 104
bias, 49, 55, 61

bilateral, 132, 154, 155
biomarkers, 8, 14
biomonitoring, 129
biosensors, 34
bleeding, 20, 22
bleeding time, 20
blood, vii, ix, 2, 4, 5, 6, 8, 9, 10, 11, 12, 15, 16, 20, 21, 24, 82, 83, 84, 104, 113, 115, 129, 136, 139, 140, 141
blood circulation, 141
blood clot, 17
blood flow, 17, 139
blood pressure reduction, 5, 9, 11
blood stream, 20
blood vessels, 21
bloodstream, 140
Bluetooth, 117, 121, 123, 124, 125
body weight, 9
bone, 149
brain, ix, 27, 29, 31, 32, 34, 46, 72, 110, 133, 136, 137, 138, 139, 140, 141, 142, 143, 146, 150, 151, 153, 154, 155, 157, 158
brain activity, 32
brain functions, 136
brain stem, 136
brain structure, 133, 142
brainstem, 136
brainstorming, 30
breastfeeding, 144
breathing, vii, 22, 23
breathing rate, vii
bronchioles, 23
Brownian motion, 139

C

calibration, 47, 53, 82, 95, 97, 103, 104, 128
cancer, 9, 11
candidates, 144, 145
car accidents, 108

car drivers, 108
carbon, 20
carbon dioxide, 20
cardiac activity, 46
cardiac output, 84
cardiac surgery, 85
cardiovascular disease, ix, 2, 9, 13, 108
cardiovascular risk, 7
case study, 69
central nervous system (CNS), 21
cerebellum, 136
cerebral blood flow, 139
cerebral cortex, 132, 136
cerebral hemisphere, 136
cerebrospinal fluid, 136, 150
cerebrum, 136
challenges, 104
Chicago, 73
children, 3, 158
China, 74, 130, 144
classes, 29, 36, 38, 40, 58, 59, 60, 61, 64, 65, 66, 67, 68
classification, 28, 33, 36, 37, 38, 40, 41, 42, 48, 57, 58, 59, 60, 62, 63, 64, 68
clinical depression, 131, 132, 135
clothing, 24, 47
clustering, 48
clusters, 151
coefficient of variation, 36
cognitive function, 29
cognitive impairment, 131
coherence, 39, 139
collaboration, 88
color, 22, 93, 153
communication, 46, 48, 49, 85, 86, 105, 114, 117, 124, 125, 127
community, 132
compatibility, 49
complexity, 71, 144
compliance, 5
complications, 15, 16, 17, 23, 112

composition, 9
computer, 2, 73
computer use, 2
computing, 39, 75
connectivity, x, 132, 133, 137, 138, 139, 141, 142, 143, 151, 154, 155, 157, 158
consciousness, 84, 136
Consensus, 13
consumption, 119, 128
continuous exercise, 2, 5, 6, 8, 9, 12
coordination, 136
coronary artery disease, 4
coronary heart disease, 10, 12
corpus callosum, 136, 154
correlation, 37, 82, 138, 141, 150, 156, 157
correlation coefficient, 150
correlations, x, 132
cortex, 17, 136, 138, 139, 153
cortical volume, x, 132, 142, 150, 151, 152, 153, 155
cost, x, 46, 52, 59, 71, 87, 104, 115, 118, 123, 126, 138
cough, 23
counseling, 133
credentials, 84, 98
cyanosis, 22, 23

D

danger, 86
data analysis, 111
data collection, 88
data distribution, 64
data mining, 73
database, 40, 55, 112, 141
Decision Trees, 28, 57, 58, 68
decomposition, 36, 71
deep learning, 73
deformation, 61
dehydration, 24
delirium, 24

Delta, 51
delusions, 134
dementia, 29
denoising, 41
Department of Transportation, 128
depressants, 20
depression, 21, 30, 131, 132, 133, 134, 135, 141, 142, 145, 153, 155, 156, 157, 158, 159
deprivation, 23
depth, 20, 76, 77
detection, ix, 28, 31, 32, 33, 34, 35, 36, 37, 38, 40, 41, 42, 46, 48, 53, 55, 56, 57, 59, 64, 65, 66, 67, 68, 69, 70, 72, 73, 74, 75, 76, 77, 78, 92, 95, 108, 111, 116, 127, 128, 154
detection system, 28, 42, 53, 55, 59, 74, 76, 77
deviation, 38, 39
diabetes, 108, 109
diabetes disease, 108
Diagnostic and Statistical Manual of Mental Disorders, 135
diastolic pressure, 82
diffusion, 138, 157
digestion, 136
dimensionality, 48
disability, 19, 132, 158
Discriminant Analysis, 28, 38, 39, 41, 57, 59, 68
diseases, ix, 1, 2, 4, 29, 141, 158
disorder, 27, 28, 29, 131, 133, 134, 142, 155
displacement, 95
distracters, 159
distribution, 35, 59, 77
diversity, 58, 111
doctors, 122
DOI, 7, 8, 9, 10, 11, 12, 13
dopaminergic, 30
doppler, 75, 76
dose-response relationship, 1, 4
drug delivery, 83

drug flow, 86
drug library, 82, 84, 86, 87, 99, 100, 104
drugs, 20, 83, 85, 87, 99, 100, 104, 144
DS-1, 91

E

ECG, ix, 28, 32, 36, 40, 41, 46, 47, 48, 49, 50, 51, 52, 54, 55, 66, 67, 68, 84, 90, 91, 100, 101, 102, 112, 113, 114, 115, 129
education, 19
EEG, ix, 28, 32, 34, 35, 36, 37, 38, 39, 40, 41, 46, 47, 48, 49, 50, 51, 54, 55, 67, 68, 69, 70, 71, 72, 73, 84, 140
electrodes, 32, 47, 48, 50, 91, 100, 101, 113, 114, 115, 129, 140
electroencephalogram, 72
electroencephalography, 73
electrolyte, 16, 23
electrolyte imbalance, 23
electrophysiological signals, 28
e-mail, 19
emergency, 31, 32, 108, 117, 127, 128
emotion, 159
emotional disorder, 134
emotional health, 135
empathy, 153, 158
employees, 6
encouragement, 19
endocrine, ix, 15, 16, 18
energy, 2, 3, 4, 35, 36, 37, 39, 138, 141
energy expenditure, 2, 4
engineering, vii, x, 73, 74, 75, 86
Ensemble Learning, 28, 57, 63, 64, 65, 68
entropy, 38, 39, 74
environment, x, 23, 24, 30, 49, 77, 82, 88, 115, 123
epidemiology, 1, 4
epilepsy, 28, 29, 30, 31, 34, 36, 37, 38, 41, 42, 45, 46, 48, 60, 65, 66, 68, 69, 71, 72
epileptic seizure, 28, 35, 37, 38, 39, 40, 41, 42, 57, 69, 71, 72, 73
epinephrine, 16
equilibrium, 150
equipment, 108
evidence, 4
evil, 134
evolution, 30, 35
exercise, ix, 2, 3, 4, 5, 6, 7, 8, 9, 10, 11, 12, 13
extraction, x, 73
extracts, 38

F

false alarms, 108, 110, 118, 127
families, 45
fat, 6, 21
fear, 18, 19, 21
features extraction, 37, 50
feelings, 131, 135, 136
fever, 23, 24
field theory, 151
filters, 35, 37, 126
first aid, 34
fitness, 3, 5, 7, 8, 9, 12, 13
flow rate, 82, 83, 103
fluctuations, 139
fluid, 16, 23, 137
fMRI, 139, 140, 141, 142, 146, 156, 157, 158
force, 105, 109, 128
forecasting, 48
frontal cortex, 153, 155
frontal lobe, 136, 153
functional analysis, 146, 155
functional connectivity, x, 132, 133, 138, 139, 141, 142, 143, 151, 154, 155, 157
Functional Magnetic Resonance Imaging (fMRI), 157, 158
functional MRI, 150

G

gel, 100
general adaptation syndrome, 16
general anesthesia, 20, 21
generalized seizures, 29
gland, 17
glasses, 112
glucocorticoid, 17
glucose, 17, 128
Google, 52, 54
GPS, 46
gravity, 29, 30, 77
gray matter, 136, 149, 150, 156
grounding, 47
group variance, 151
grouping, 123
growth, 23, 155
Guangzhou, 130
guidance, 8
guidelines, 2, 99
guilty, 136

H

hallucinations, 134
hazards, 29
healing, 19
health, vii, x, 1, 2, 3, 4, 6, 7, 8, 11, 19, 29, 30, 42, 69, 74, 77, 84, 108, 110, 111, 113, 114, 117, 119, 121, 127, 129, 142, 157
health care, vii, x, 108, 110, 117, 119, 121, 127
health care professionals, 110, 117
health condition, 3, 4, 84, 129
health problems, vii, 30, 108, 110, 127
health status, 111
heart attack, 109
heart disease, 13, 109
heart rate, x, 16, 20, 21, 52, 55, 66, 83, 91, 108, 114, 122
height, 101
hemisphere, 150, 153
heterogeneity, 35
history, 77
homeostasis, 19
hopelessness, 134
hormone, 17
hormones, 16
hospitalization, 7
host, 90
human, x, 74, 75, 77, 78, 87, 135, 136, 137, 138, 141, 157
human brain, 136, 137, 141, 157
humidity, 92, 101
hybrid, 74
hypertension, 4, 7, 8, 11, 12
hyperthermia, 23
hypotension, 4, 5
hypothalamus, 16
hypothermia, 22
hypothesis, 146
hypoxia, 21, 23

I

ICE, 121
identification, 73
image, 77, 97, 137, 142, 145, 147, 149
images, 76, 139, 140, 141, 142, 145, 147, 149, 156, 157
incidence, 1, 2, 5, 6, 87, 133, 158
income, 30
independence, 139
India, 34, 69, 78, 128
individuals, 6, 16, 30, 31, 135
inefficiency, 84
infection, 23, 24
inflammation, 5

Information and Communication Technologies, 76
information technology, 74
injuries, 158
injury, iv
input signal, 50
insulation, 21
insulin, 5
insulin sensitivity, 5
integration, ix, 83, 84, 104, 137, 141
integrity, 111, 154, 159
intelligent ICU, 82
intensive care unit, 82, 83, 87, 105, 106
interdependence, 139
interface, 50, 54, 94, 96, 117
interference, 44, 50, 52, 76, 126
intermittent exercise, 2, 5, 6
international standards, 83
intravenously, 83, 140
inventions, 104
inversion, 39
issues, 109, 110, 111

K

kidney, 17
KNN, 28, 37, 38, 41, 43, 44, 57, 62, 63, 64, 68, 74

L

laser ablation, 34
latency, 35, 42
lead, 17, 29, 47, 85, 87, 131, 132, 155
learners, 63
learning, 19, 30, 36, 40, 49, 55, 63, 72
learning difficulties, 30
Lebanon, 1, 27, 81, 107, 131
leisure, 3, 11
lethargy, 16

life cycle, 111
lifetime, 133
light, 24, 107, 115, 126, 155
linear model, 151
linen, 24
lipemia, 5, 12
lipids, 12
living conditions, 30
localization, 140
location detection, 108
logging, 101
lying, 2

M

machine learning, 32, 35, 38, 46, 72, 156
magnet, 142
magnetic field, 140, 142
magnetic properties, 142
magnetic resonance, 136, 140, 144, 158
magnetic resonance image, 158
magnetic resonance imaging, 136, 140, 144
magnetization, 150
magnitude, 2
major depression, 142, 159
major depressive disorder, x, 132, 134, 135, 142, 155, 158
major issues, 46
majority, 21, 64, 135
mammalian brain, 139
management, 23, 85, 129
manifolds, 77
manipulation, 46
manufacturing, 104
mapping, 144
Markov chain, 44
mass, 5, 114
matrix, 59, 145
matter, 136, 137, 139, 150, 154
measurement, vii, 19, 53, 91, 108, 111, 112, 113, 121

Index

measurements, ix, x, 6, 28, 74, 88, 95, 100, 104, 112, 115, 116, 126, 141, 151
medical, x, 22, 31, 82, 83, 84, 86, 87, 88, 98, 99, 104, 105, 108, 109, 110, 111, 115, 118, 122, 125, 127, 132, 135
medical assistance, 31
medical care, 22
medication, 49, 82, 85, 86, 87, 105, 133, 144, 153
medicine, 74
medulla, 16, 136
memory, 29, 104, 120, 153
memory loss, 29
mental health, 3, 134, 135
mental illness, 135
messages, 136
meta-analysis, 7, 8, 9, 12, 13
metabolic syndrome, 6
meter, 138
methodology, 143
microcontroller, 46, 50, 68, 82, 93, 111, 112, 118, 120, 124
Microsoft, 49
Minneapolis, 106
misuse, 108
mobile device, 50
mobile phone, 32, 46, 50, 52, 54
models, 48, 59, 76, 108
modifications, 115
modules, 90
molecules, 139
momentum, 55
mood disorder, 132, 142
morbidity, 87, 104
morphological variations, 138
morphometric, x, 132, 143
mortality, ix, 1, 2, 4, 6, 7, 9, 10, 11, 13, 85, 87, 104, 110
mortality rate, 85, 104
motor control, 140
mucus, 23
muscle atrophy, 29

N

narcotics, 23
National Health and Nutrition Examination Survey, 13
negative emotions, 153
nerve, 136
neural networks, 38, 46
neural systems, 74
neurobiology, 156
neurodegenerative diseases, 31
neurodegenerative disorders, 29, 30
neuroimaging, 133, 146
neurological disease, 138
neurological disorder, 27, 28
neuromotor, 8
neurons, 29, 55, 56, 136, 138
neuroscience, 105
next generation, 86
norepinephrine, 16
normal aging, 159
null, 104
nurses, x, 82, 83, 86, 87, 88, 98
nursing, ix, 16, 17, 22, 23, 82, 83, 86
nursing care, ix, 16, 82

O

obstacles, 115
occipital lobe, 136
occlusion, 77
operating system, 48
opioids, 20
opportunities, 30
optimization, 49, 55, 56, 61, 67
organism, 16
outpatient, 144
overweight, 12
ox, 115
oxidative stress, 5
oxygen, 20, 82, 84, 91, 115, 140

P

pain, ix, 10, 15, 16, 19, 24
pallor, 22
parallel, 32
paralysis, 29
parasympathetic activity, 5
parents, 46
parietal lobe, 136
participants, x, 1, 4, 8
pathogenesis, 132
pathophysiology, 154
pathway, 139
patient care, 17
pattern recognition, 75
peace, 45
personal life, 142
phone application, 30, 32, 46, 48, 50, 52, 54, 108, 110, 111, 119, 121, 123, 125, 127
physical activity, ix, 1, 2, 3, 6, 7, 8, 10, 11, 12, 13, 14
physical fitness, 3, 7
physical inactivity, ix, 1, 2, 9
physicians, 88
physics, 73, 75
physiological patient monitor, 82, 85
pituitary gland, 16
plasma levels, 24
platform, 77, 93, 105
pneumonia, 23
Poincaré, 72
population, 2, 8, 142
positive correlation, 2
pregnancy, 144
premature death, 2, 4, 30
preparation, 15, 19, 24
prevention, ix, 1, 3, 4, 7, 10
primary function, 24
principal component analysis, 78
probability, 58, 110, 148

profit, 83
programming, 86, 100, 104, 123
project, 28, 32, 39, 41, 45, 57, 68, 109, 127, 128, 132
propagation, 49
protection, 128, 137
prototype, 67, 90, 93, 95, 96, 97, 100, 104
psychiatric disorder, 131
psychoanalysis, 135
psychological well-being, 18
public health, x, 6, 9, 69
pulmonary embolism, 24
pumps, 84, 86, 87, 88, 104, 106, 115

Q

qualifications, 87
quality of life, 3, 30
query, 123
questionnaire, 135

R

radar, 75
radio, 117, 142
Ramadan, 9
reactions, 18, 88, 109
reading, 47, 91, 99, 111, 120, 126
real time, 92
reasoning, 74
recognition, 1, 2, 140
recommendations, iv, 3
reconstruction, 139, 158
recovery, 20, 21, 82
redundancy, 111
regression, 41, 48, 60, 157
regression method, 60
rehabilitation, 74
relatives, 144
relaxation, 149

relaxation times, 149
reliability, 111, 112, 127, 128
renin, 5
requirements, 19, 83, 111, 115, 118
researchers, 30, 34, 35, 37, 40, 41, 42, 112, 113, 138, 146, 156
resistance, 5
resolution, x, 41, 73, 132, 138
respiration, 17, 20
respiratory rate, ix, 15, 16
response, 2, 8, 13, 16, 24, 58, 59, 112, 115, 158
response time, 112, 115
restoration, 30
risk, 1, 2, 4, 5, 6, 8, 11, 13, 18, 23, 30, 31, 82, 83, 85, 111, 127, 142
risk factors, 5, 13
risks, vii, ix, 29, 47
ROI, x, 132, 139, 141, 147, 150
room temperature, 21, 92, 101
root, 58
rules, 39, 49, 72, 130

S

sadness, 131, 132, 135
safe system, 108, 161
safety, 34, 68, 83, 88, 99, 104, 105, 109, 110, 111, 118, 127, 128
sample mean, 59
saturation, 20, 84, 91
school, 30
science, 13, 73
scientific papers, 113
sedentary behavior, 2, 10
seed, x, 132, 141, 150, 155, 157
segregation, 137
seizure, x, 28, 31, 32, 34, 35, 36, 37, 38, 39, 40, 41, 46, 48, 49, 50, 57, 64, 69, 70, 71, 72, 73
self-esteem, 134

self-monitoring, 34
sensations, 29
sensing, 129
sensitivity, 28, 35, 36, 37, 38, 40, 41, 42, 57, 64, 65, 66, 68, 115, 117
sensor, 37, 43, 44, 46, 48, 67, 75, 76, 91, 92, 108, 110, 111, 112, 113, 115, 118, 120, 121, 123, 124, 126, 128
sensor network, 37, 75
sensors, 31, 32, 34, 37, 42, 43, 44, 46, 48, 52, 53, 68, 75, 76, 97, 99, 101, 108, 110, 112, 113, 114, 115, 116, 118, 121, 123, 124, 125, 126, 128, 129
services, iv, 82
shape, 30, 77, 78
shock, 137
shortage, 83, 104
showing, x, 48, 57, 97, 99, 119, 132, 137, 141, 143, 152
signals, 28, 32, 35, 36, 37, 40, 46, 48, 49, 50, 55, 90, 100, 101, 102, 112, 114, 136, 141
signs, vii, ix, x, 15, 16, 19, 22, 23, 24, 28, 30, 33, 46, 86, 87, 108, 109, 110, 112, 113, 114, 118, 127, 128, 129
silhouette, 77
simulation, 33, 40, 57, 86, 88
skeletal muscle, 4
skin, 17, 19, 21, 22, 100
sleep deprivation, 23
smart syringe pump, x, 82, 86
smoothing, 36, 147, 149
SMS, 110, 112, 121
social activities, 30
society, 31, 32, 133
sodium, 17
software, 48, 54, 84, 87, 93, 105, 110, 118, 119, 124, 126, 144, 149, 151
solution, 30, 82, 85, 87, 96, 108
spin, 149
spinal cord, 136, 137
SPO2, x, 108, 110, 115, 116, 120, 122, 123

Spring, 73
sputum, 24
sputum culture, 24
stability, 22, 30
standard deviation, 37, 51, 55
stasis, 17
state, 19, 21, 33, 35, 40, 44, 46, 49, 52, 59, 114, 121, 127, 128, 140, 157
states, 1, 2, 33, 67, 71, 140
statistics, 139
stimulation, 16, 21
stimulus, 140
storage, 104, 120
stress, ix, 8, 15, 16, 17, 18, 29
stress reactions, 18
stressors, 16
structural changes, x, 132
structural characteristics, 144
structural connectivity, 132, 133, 138, 142, 151, 158
structure, 43, 136
style, vii
suicide, 142
supervisor, 32
suppression, 76
surface area, x, 132, 142, 151, 152, 153, 155, 159
surgical resection, 34
surgical stress, ix, 16, 18
surveillance, 8, 77
Sustainable Development, 2
SVM, 28, 35, 36, 37, 38, 39, 40, 41, 43, 44, 57, 60, 61, 62, 68, 70
sympathetic nervous system, 16
symptoms, 16, 27, 29, 132, 134, 135
synaptic strength, 138
synchronization, 39, 71
systolic blood pressure, 4
systolic pressure, 82

T

tachycardia, 23
tachypnea, 23
Taiwan, 129
target, 2, 108, 111, 128
teams, 83
techniques, 20, 63, 141, 143, 156
technologies, 82, 104
technology, 86, 117, 129, 142
television viewing, 2
temperature, vii, 16, 20, 21, 24, 84, 92, 101
temporal lobe, 71, 136
temporal lobe epilepsy, 71
testing, 33, 36, 48, 49, 55, 56, 60, 62, 64, 68, 96, 119, 127, 128
therapy, 132
thermoregulation, 21
thrombophlebitis, 24
time series, 132, 141, 150
tissue, 16, 139, 148
topology, 61
training, ix, 5, 12, 36, 55, 56, 58, 60, 61, 62, 63, 64, 67, 88
transactions, 74
transducer, 44
transformation, 150
transmission, 47
trauma, 15, 17, 144
treatment, ix, x, 1, 3, 4, 31, 82, 88, 133, 135, 154, 156
trial, 48
triceps, 6
Turkey, 15
type 2 diabetes, 12

U

unhappiness, 134
United States, 10, 133, 135

urethra, 17
urinary tract, 24
urinary tract infection, 24
urine, 17, 24

V

validation, 40, 110, 126
valueless, 136
variables, 114, 141
variations, 20, 139, 155, 156
vasoconstriction, 17
vector, 38, 44, 61, 71, 77, 78
vehicles, 109
velocity, 76
vessels, 17
vibration, 43, 76, 126
videos, 77
vision, 156
visualization, 96
vital signs, vii, ix, x, 15, 16, 19, 22, 23, 24, 28, 33, 46, 86, 87, 108, 109, 110, 112, 113, 114, 118, 127, 128, 129
vital signs measurement, 108, 112
voting, 61, 64

W

waking, 2

walking, 10, 11
war, 130
Washington, 128
watches, 112
water, 17, 139
wavelet, 36, 37, 38, 39, 51, 70, 71, 75
wavelet analysis, 71
weight loss, 12
well-being, 3
wellness, 132
white matter, 136, 137, 139, 149, 150, 153, 159
Wi-Fi, 49
wires, 47
work activities, 28
workers, 7
workflow, 88
workforce, 31
working memory, 159
workload, 16, 83, 86, 98
World Health Organization, 30, 69, 132
worldwide, 29, 30, 131
worry, 135

Y

yield, vii